THE SLOW COOKER COOKBOOK

THE SLOW COOKER COOKBOOK

75 Easy, Healthy, and Delicious Recipes for Slow-Cooked Meals

SALINAS PRESS

Copyright © 2013 by Salinas Press, Berkeley, California

No part of this publication may be reproduced, stored in a retrieval system or transmitted in any form or by any means, electronic, mechanical, photocopying, recording, scanning or otherwise, except as permitted under Sections 107 or 108 of the 1976 United States Copyright Act, without the prior written permission of the Publisher. Requests to the Publisher for permission should be addressed to the Permissions Department, Salinas Press, 918 Parker St, Suite A-12, Berkeley, CA 94710.

Limit of Liability/Disclaimer of Warranty: The Publisher and the author make no representations or warranties with respect to the accuracy or completeness of the contents of this work and specifically disclaim all warranties, including without limitation warranties of fitness for a particular purpose. No warranty may be created or extended by sales or promotional materials. The advice and strategies contained herein may not be suitable for every situation. This work is sold with the understanding that the publisher is not engaged in rendering medical, legal or other professional advice or services. If professional assistance is required, the services of a competent professional person should be sought. Neither the Publisher nor the author shall be liable for damages arising herefrom. The fact that an individual, organization or website is referred to in this work as a citation and/or potential source of further information does not mean that the author or the Publisher endorses the information the individual, organization or website may provide or recommendations they/it may make. Further, readers should be aware that Internet websites listed in this work may have changed or disappeared between when this work was written and when it is read.

For general information on our other products and services or to obtain technical support, please contact our Customer Care Department within the U.S. at (866) 744-2665, or outside the U.S. at (510) 253-0500.

Salinas Press publishes its books in a variety of electronic and print formats. Some content that appears in print may not be available in electronic books, and vice versa.

TRADEMARKS: Salinas Press and the Salinas Press logo are trademarks or registered trademarks of Callisto Media Inc. and/or its affiliates, in the United States and other countries, and may not be used without written permission. All other trademarks are the property of their respective owners. Salinas Press is not associated with any product or vendor mentioned in this book.

ISBN: Print 978-1-62315-163-8 | eBook 978-1-62315-164-5

Contents

CHAPTER ONE
The Basics

What Is the Difference Between a Crock Pot and a Slow Cooker?   4
Basics of Slow Cooker Cooking   4
Two Types of Slow Cooker Cooking   4
The Basics of a Slow Cooker Pantry   5
Cooking Methods   7
Before You Begin   8

CHAPTER TWO
What's for Breakfast?

Classic Strata   14
Sausage and Potato Casserole   15
Spicy Pears with Cranberries   16
Slow Cooker Oatmeal   17

CHAPTER THREE
Soups and Stews

Baked Potato Soup   22
Multi-Mushroom Soup   23
Slow-Cooked Butternut Squash Soup   24
Roasted Tomato Soup   25
Cream of Broccoli Soup   26
Ham and White Bean Soup   27

Hearty Bean Soup   28
Chicken and Wild Rice Soup   29
Spicy Chicken Tortilla Soup   30
Summer Vegetable Soup   31

CHAPTER FOUR

American Favorites

Old-Fashioned Beef Stew   36
Shredded Buffalo Chicken   37
Pulled-Pork Barbecue   38
Old-Fashioned Meatloaf   39
Barbecued Baby Back Ribs   40
Pork Chops with Apples and Sauerkraut   41
Franks and Beans   42
Chicken Potpie   43
Classic Pot Roast   44

CHAPTER FIVE

International Dishes

Tandoori Chicken   48
Moroccan Chicken Tagine   49
Miso Chicken with Broccoli   50
North African Beef Stew   51
Osso Bucco   52
Curried Coconut Chicken with Basil   53
Kielbasa and Sauerkraut   54
Veal Paprikash   55
Mexican-Style Pork   56
Braised Asian Beef   57
Mediterranean Lamb   58

CHAPTER SIX
Fish and Seafood

Bouillabaisse 62
Poached Tuna 64
Lemon and Garlic Halibut 65
Sweet Miso-Glazed Cod 66
Poached Salmon Cakes with White Wine Butter Sauce 67
Sea Bass with Spicy Crusted Potatoes 68
Green Curried Shrimp 69

CHAPTER SEVEN
Casseroles

Tuna Noodle Casserole 74
Classic Lasagna Bolognese 75
Salmon, Artichoke, and Noodle Casserole 77
Chicken and Mushroom Casserole 78

CHAPTER EIGHT
Sides and Starters

Southern-Style Green Beans 82
Orange-Glazed Carrots 83
Braised Root Vegetables 84
Tomatoes, Corn, and Yellow Squash with Herbed Butter 85
Caribbean Black Beans 86
Roasted Beets with Pomegranate Dressing 87
Garlic and Rosemary Red Potatoes 88
Polenta 89
Risotto alla Milanese 90
Saffron Rice 91

Fruited Wild Rice Pilaf   92
Classic Bread Stuffing   93
Cornbread Stuffing   94
Vegetarian Cassoulet   95
Eggplant Parmesan   97
Zucchini, Leek, and Tomato Gratin   98
Ratatouille with Goat Cheese and Basil   99
Italian Cocktail Meatballs   100
Asian Honey Chicken Wings   101
Super Bowl Chili   102

CHAPTER NINE

Desserts and Drinks

Strawberry Rhubarb White Chocolate Crumble   106
Spiced Pear Crumble   107
Apple Cranberry Cobbler   108
Hot Fudge Cake   109
Chocolate Croissant Bread Pudding   110
Tapioca Pudding   111
Wassail   112
Warmed Cranberry Punch   113
Wild Chocolate Mocha   114
Creamy Hot Cocoa   115

Index   116

CHAPTER ONE

The Basics

CHAPTER ONE

The Basics

When you think about slow cookers, what comes to mind? If you answered hearty winter meals such as savory stews or pot roasts, you are not alone. For many, this is the only type of food for which they use their slow cookers. If you love stews and pot roasts, that's great, but what if you are looking for something different?

You don't have to look anymore. Cooking in a slow cooker can be easy, fun, and delicious. It's something that you can do on a daily basis to get dinner on the table—even if that dinner is a sharp and cheesy lasagna or a light and flavorful salmon chowder. You can make just about anything in a slow cooker, and in this book, you'll be amazed by recipes you'd never dreamed you could prepare so easily, ranging from breakfasts to desserts (yes, dessert!).

WHAT IS THE DIFFERENCE BETWEEN A CROCK POT AND A SLOW COOKER?

There is no difference, except that the term "Crock Pot" is a trademark owned by Rival; they invented the concept of a slow cooker back in the '70s. They are the same thing—a pot with high and low settings that cooks for long periods of time at a low temperature.

BASICS OF SLOW COOKER COOKING

So, first up, what is a slow cooker, and who would want to use it? Well, truth be told, it's one of the simplest appliances in your kitchen. It might also be the one that will get the most use if you know how to use it correctly—which you will after you have read this book.

With just two settings, high and low, a slow cooker works its magic by transforming the ingredients you throw into the pot into a yummy meal at a slow and steady pace. In fact, even the high setting is not really high; it's around 300 degrees Fahrenheit, which is pretty low compared to typical oven settings. But this is where the slow cooker shines. It works by heating foods at a low temperature for a long period of time, with the end result being tender meats, flavorful vegetables, and delectable dishes that benefit from all those aromas being trapped in that pot for hours at a time.

Who has eight hours to wait for dinner to be ready? Everyone, including you. You're at work all day, right? If so, you are the person for whom the slow cooker was invented. Unlike traditional cooking in which you have to spend an hour or so in the kitchen preparing your meal, the slow cooker works while you do. You simply get it started in the morning, and when you come home, your dinner is ready. No more getting home after a long day and wondering what you're going to do for dinner. You can eat immediately upon arrival and spend the rest of your evening doing what you enjoy. You won't even have a lot of dishes to wash because, for the most part, your meal was cooked in one pot.

TWO TYPES OF SLOW COOKER COOKING

There are two types of slow cooker cooking; one is easier than the other, although neither is really difficult. However, the end results will be much different.

The first method is the easiest, and one that you may rely on when you want the simplest way of cooking possible. You put everything in the pot—meat, vegetables, and rice—cover it, turn it on, and go. After eight hours, you come home to a meal, with virtually no cleanup.

The other method is similar, except that you prepare some of the ingredients in another pan—for example, browning meats or sautéing vegetables—before throwing them in the cooker.

Why would you want to use the second method, since it is obviously more trouble than the first? The reason is pure and simple: flavor. The slow cooker will tenderize the roast and soften up the vegetables, but there is nothing quite like the aroma and flavor you get from a good browned crust on a pot roast.

While the recipes in this book usually give you instructions for the second method of cooking, feel free to skip the preparation steps and throw your ingredients into the pot as is. All of the recipes in this book work either way.

Before you get started, there are several things that will make using a slow cooker more enjoyable and give you better results; this is the easiest form of cooking you'll ever do, but it doesn't hurt to know a bit before you begin.

THE BASICS OF A SLOW COOKER PANTRY

You can use a slow cooker for just about any meal. It's great to have when you know you'll have a busy day and want to have dinner ready when you get home.

Keep these items on hand, and you'll be able to put together a delicious meal at a moment's notice.

Refrigerated Items

- Unsalted butter
- Heavy cream
- Cheese
- Whole milk
- Fruit
- Fresh lemons, oranges, and limes
- Fresh herbs to add at the end of cooking

Frozen Items*

- Meats, such as frozen chicken breasts, roasts, and pork chops
- An assortment of fruits and vegetables

* Do not put any frozen food in your cooker, including vegetables. They will reduce the temperature of the cooker and add extra moisture. Always thaw ingredients before use.

Canned Goods

- Beans
- Tomatoes
- Tomato paste
- Chicken, beef, and vegetable broth
- Canned chilies
- Prepared salsa

Oil/Vinegar/Flavoring

- Vegetable oil, for sautéing foods when you don't want to add a lot of flavor
- Olive oil, for adding a depth of flavor to certain dishes
- Sesame oil, for Asian dishes
- Balsamic vinegar
- Apple cider vinegar
- Red wine vinegar
- Soy sauce
- Mustard
- Tabasco or your favorite hot sauce

Starches

- Hard durum wheat pastas, which are best for the slow cooker
- Brown, white, wild, arborio, and jasmine rices
- Grains such as barley, bulgur, and millet
- Dried beans, peas, and lentils

Dried Herbs and Spices

- Allspice
- Basil
- Bay leaves (always remove these before serving, as they can be a choking hazard)
- Cayenne pepper
- Chili powder
- Cinnamon (both ground and whole sticks)
- Cloves
- Coriander
- Cumin (ground)

- Curry powder
- Fennel seeds
- Herbs de Provence
- Jerk seasoning
- Marjoram
- Powdered mustard
- Nutmeg
- Oregano
- Paprika
- Rosemary
- Saffron (it's expensive, but a little goes a long way)
- Sage
- Thyme

COOKING METHODS

You'll find that while you can cook almost anything in a slow cooker, some foods work better than others. The following foods can be put in the cooker and will be tender and delicious after an eight-hour slow braise:

- Tough cuts of meat such as whole chuck roasts, pork roasts, chicken breasts and thighs, lamb, and veal
- Hearty vegetables, including potatoes, carrots, turnips, beets, and celery
- Greens, including spinach, kale, collards, and mustard greens
- Cabbage, broccoli, and cauliflower
- Beans and lentils

Some foods will not be able to withstand that much cooking. The following list contains foods that either need a much shorter cooking time or must be added near the end of the cycle:

- Dairy products such as milk, yogurt, and sour cream, all of which should be added just before serving or they are likely to curdle. Some dairy products may be added in the beginning but cooked on the low setting.
- Fresh herbs, which should be added in the last 15 minutes of cook time, with the exception of rosemary, which can be added at the beginning
- Seafood and shellfish, which will overcook if left for too long and become chewy and rubbery

The key to excellent results in your slow cooker is to experiment and use common sense. By doing so, you'll soon be creating amazing recipes on your own, and your slow cooker will become one of your favorite cooking appliances.

BEFORE YOU BEGIN

- Slow cookers come in a variety of sizes, and, yes, size does matter. If you don't already have one, you should ask yourself how many people you are going to feed on a regular basis, and buy accordingly. For the best results, you do not want to fill the pot less than half or more than three-quarters full. This means if you buy an extra-large pot, you'll be making extra-large amounts of food. If you're not sure what capacity to get, or you think you will alternate the amount of food you cook in it, get two. They're not that expensive, and the quality of your dishes will be worth it. On average, a four- to five-quart slow cooker will generously feed a family of four. This is the size of the slow cooker that will be used for the recipes in this book, unless otherwise noted.
- There are only two settings on a slow cooker: high and low. The low setting is what you'll use if you plan on leaving for an entire day (eight hours or more) and want to have dinner ready when you come home. You can cut your time by about half with the high setting; in general, one hour on high equals two hours on low. While some cookers have extra features such as timers and warming functions, all you need for fabulous meals are those two settings: high and low.
- The cooker has a lid, and this is one of the fundamentals of slow cooking. When you put a lid on the pot, you are trapping in the steam and aroma of your dish. You should not take the lid off unless instructed to do so in the recipe, and even then, only when necessary. Removing it before the dish is finished will result in a much longer cooking time, and possibly the loss of flavor.
- Do not put frozen foods in a slow cooker; in fact, it's best if all food is at room temperature. Remember, a cooker does not get super hot, so adding cold foods will dramatically slow down an already lengthy process.
- Some foods should not go in until near the end. Fish and shellfish, dairy products, and fresh herbs will not benefit from extra-long cooking time, no matter how low the temperature. Shorter cooking times (four hours) on low are usually okay. Dried herbs, on the other hand, are fine to simmer in a sauce for hours. To liven it up, simply add fresh herbs near the end.
- The order in which the ingredients go into the pot is important, so when following the recipes in this book, make sure to pay attention to the correct order. In general, extremely dense foods such as potatoes or root vegetables that take the longest to cook will go on the bottom, with lighter ingredients on top.
- When chopping and prepping vegetables and other ingredients, cut them to the same size to ensure that everything is cooked evenly.

- You don't have to brown meat before cooking it in a slow cooker, but if you sear it with a little oil in a skillet, the meat will have a more complex flavor. Always brown any ground meat before adding it to a slow cooker, otherwise the meat will clump and add too much grease to the dish.
- Like most cooking, slow cooking is not an exact science. Many things will affect the results of your dish, even if you follow the recipes exactly. Just as every vegetable and piece of meat is not exactly the same, neither will be the results of your meal. Don't worry. If you follow the directions and keep the general principles of a slow cooker in mind, you will have no problems. Just be aware that sometimes you'll need to make adjustments.

So now that we've got the basics out of the way, there's nothing left to do but get started making delicious recipes.

CHAPTER TWO

What's for Breakfast?

CHAPTER TWO

What's for Breakfast?

You can use a slow cooker for anything, including breakfast. It's easy to have a hearty breakfast when you just put the ingredients in the cooker and go to bed. When you wake up in the morning, you'll have a delicious hot breakfast waiting for you.

You can also use the cooker for brunch, easily crossing one more thing off your list.

Classic Strata

SERVES 8

With layers of eggs and bread, this makes a hearty meal that is perfect for brunch or early-morning company. This recipe is pretty basic, but feel free to add whatever you like to the mix. Vegetables, herbs, and spices all work well here. Use your imagination and you'll be creating new favorites before you know it.

6 CUPS TORN BREAD, PREFERABLY STALE
3 CUPS SHREDDED CHEDDAR CHEESE
3 CUPS MILK
6 EGGS
2 DROPS HOT SAUCE
SALT, TO TASTE

Grease the inside of the slow cooker with cooking spray, butter, or oil.

Cover the bottom of the cooker with 2 cups of bread. Sprinkle with 1 cup of cheese. Repeat with a second layer of bread, a second layer of cheese, and then a third layer of bread. Reserve the remaining cup of cheese.

Whisk the milk, eggs, and hot sauce with a pinch of salt. Pour into the slow cooker, and push it down to make sure it becomes saturated. Sprinkle the remaining cup of cheese on top.

Cover and cook on low for 4 hours, until the strata is cooked through. Remove the lid, and cook for an additional 20 minutes.

Serve warm.

Sausage and Potato Casserole

SERVES 8

This makes a delicious and filling breakfast but can also be a perfect light meal when you don't want something hearty but still want dinner ready when you get home. Feel free to add your choice of vegetables or spices to perk up this dish.

- 1 POUND BULK SAUSAGE OR COOKED OR SMOKED SAUSAGE LINKS, CUT INTO BITE-SIZED PIECES
- 1 MEDIUM ONION, CHOPPED
- 1 POUND POTATOES, SHREDDED
- 2 CUPS SHREDDED CHEDDAR CHEESE, DIVIDED
- 6 LARGE EGGS
- 1 CUP MILK
- 2 TABLESPOONS MELTED BUTTER, OPTIONAL

Grease the inside of the slow cooker with cooking spray, butter, or oil.

Add the sausage to the slow cooker along with the onion, potatoes, and 1 cup of cheese.

Whisk the eggs, milk, and butter, if using, in a medium bowl, and pour the mixture into the cooker. Cover with the rest of the cheese.

Cover and cook on high for about 3 hours until the casserole has puffed and the cheese is slightly browned.

Allow to rest for 20 minutes and serve.

Spicy Pears with Cranberries

SERVES 8

Sometimes you just want something sweet alongside your Paleo-friendly omelet. These poached pears fit the bill nicely, and they reheat well if you'd like to make a large batch to eat during the week.

8 FIRM PEARS, SUCH AS BOSC, PEELED AND CORED
½ TEASPOON GROUND CINNAMON
½ TEASPOON GROUND NUTMEG
2 TABLESPOONS COCONUT OIL
½ CUP RAW HONEY
½ TEASPOON PURE VANILLA EXTRACT
1 CUP DRIED UNSWEETENED CRANBERRIES

Cut a very thin slice from the bottom of each pear to help the fruit stand upright.

In a small dish or bowl, combine the cinnamon and nutmeg, and sprinkle the spices over the pears.

Place the pears upright in the slow cooker.

Combine the coconut oil and honey in a small saucepan. Warm over low heat just until melted. Remove from the heat and stir in the vanilla. Pour the mixture over the pears, then add cranberries to the slow cooker, distributing them evenly around the pears.

Cover and cook on low heat for 4 hours. To serve, place a pear on a small plate, spoon cranberries around it, and drizzle a little of the cooking liquid over the top.

Slow Cooker Oatmeal

SERVES 8

Nothing is better at the beginning of a long day than this hot oatmeal, cooked to perfection. It's so easy, you'll find yourself doing it often. It cooks while you sleep, allowing you to have a fast and healthful breakfast on the go.

3 CUPS ROLLED OATS (NOT THE QUICK-COOKING VARIETY)
7 CUPS WATER
PINCH OF SALT

Grease the inside of the slow cooker with cooking spray, butter, or oil.

Add the oats, water, and salt to the pot and cover. Cook on low for 8 hours.

Serve with milk, fruit, and your choice of accompaniments.

CHAPTER THREE

Soups and Stews

CHAPTER THREE

Soups and Stews

Your slow cooker is the perfect tool to create fabulous soups and stews. The long cooking time helps develop the flavor and tenderizes meats and vegetables to perfection. The recipes in this chapter are only the beginning; you can make just about any kind of soup you can imagine in a slow cooker.

Almost all of these soups can be served with crusty bread, in bread bowls, or with biscuits or cornbread. Many of them are filling enough to make a satisfying meal. You'll never buy another can of condensed soup after you see just how easy it is to make delicious homemade soups in a slow cooker.

Baked Potato Soup

SERVES 4 TO 6

This is the perfect soup to serve piping hot on a cold winter day. The combination of chicken broth and whole milk give this soup a velvety texture as well as a boost of flavor. Feel free to tweak the recipe to your liking; you can leave the skin on the potatoes or you can skip the step of pureeing the soup if you prefer a chunkier texture.

2 TABLESPOONS BUTTER, OPTIONAL
2 LARGE LEEKS, WHITE AND LIGHT GREEN PARTS, SLICED
½ TEASPOON SALT, OPTIONAL
4 LARGE RUSSET POTATOES, PEELED AND DICED
3 CUPS CHICKEN BROTH
1 CUP WHOLE MILK
SHREDDED CHEDDAR, CHOPPED GREEN ONIONS, SOUR CREAM, AND/OR CRUMBLED BACON, FOR GARNISH

Grease the inside of the slow cooker with cooking spray, butter, or oil.

If desired, sauté the leeks in the butter until tender and add them to the slow cooker. If you prefer to omit the additional fat, leave out this step and simply add the raw leeks to the slow cooker, omitting the butter. Add the salt, if using.

Add the diced potatoes to the slow cooker, followed by the chicken broth. Cover and cook on low for about 5 hours or until the potatoes are tender.

Puree the soup in batches using a blender, or use an immersion blender to puree it in the pot. Transfer back to the slow cooker, if needed, and add the milk. Cover and cook on low for 30 more minutes.

Ladle into bowls, top with desired toppings, and serve immediately.

Multi-Mushroom Soup

SERVES 4 TO 6

The flavor combination of the herbs and different types of mushrooms gives this soup an earthy flavor you'll never tire of. Choose whatever types of mushrooms you can find; the more varieties that you put in this soup, the more intense the flavor will be. Dried or fresh, either work well in this soup, so experiment until you find your perfect combination.

2 TABLESPOONS OLIVE OIL, OPTIONAL
1 MEDIUM ONION, CHOPPED
1 TEASPOON DRIED THYME OR OTHER DRIED HERBS
½ POUND SHIITAKE MUSHROOMS, SLICED
½ POUND CREMINI MUSHROOMS, SLICED
½ OUNCE DRIED PORCINI MUSHROOMS
2 TABLESPOONS SOY SAUCE
2 CUPS CHICKEN BROTH
4 SLICES BACON, COOKED AND DICED
½ CUP HALF-AND-HALF
¼ CUP MIXED FRESH HERBS (THYME, ROSEMARY, SAGE, DILL, PARSLEY, OR CHIVES IN ANY COMBINATION), CHOPPED, FOR GARNISH

Grease the inside of the slow cooker with cooking spray, butter, or oil.

For deep flavor, sauté the onion and mushrooms in the olive oil until tender. If you are pressed for time or prefer not to add extra fat, place the onion and mushrooms in the slow cooker raw and omit the olive oil.

Add the add the soy sauce, broth, and bacon to the slow cooker. Cover and cook on low for 5 to 6 hours.

Just before serving, stir in the half-and-half. Serve garnished with the fresh herbs.

Slow-Cooked Butternut Squash Soup

SERVES 4 TO 6

The bright orange squash in this soup becomes soft and sweet as it cooks down. It can be pureed for a even smoother soup if that's more your style. This soup makes an excellent starter, but if you'd rather have it as a meal, you can add crabmeat, shrimp, or chicken. If you don't want to tackle the task of cutting into a squash yourself, buy the precut variety from the produce section of your supermarket. It may cost more, but it's a great time-saver.

2 TABLESPOONS BUTTER, OPTIONAL
½ MEDIUM SWEET ONION, CHOPPED
1 MEDIUM CARROT, CHOPPED
3 CELERY STALKS, CHOPPED
1 MEDIUM BUTTERNUT SQUASH (ABOUT 2 POUNDS), PEELED AND CUBED (OR SUBSTITUTE 1½ POUNDS PRECUT SQUASH)
2 CUPS CHICKEN BROTH
1 TEASPOON DRIED THYME
SALT AND PEPPER, TO TASTE

Grease the inside of the slow cooker with cooking spray, butter, or oil.

For deep flavor, sauté the onion, carrot, and celery in the butter in a medium skillet set over medium-high heat for about 5 minutes, until the vegetables begin to soften and the onion becomes translucent. Add the cooked vegetables to the slow cooker. If you are pressed for time or prefer to skip the extra fat, you can add the vegetables directly to the slow cooker without pre-cooking, and omit the butter.

Add the squash, broth, and thyme. Season with salt and pepper.

Cover and cook on low for 5 to 6 hours. When the soup is done, puree if desired and serve.

Roasted Tomato Soup

SERVES 4 TO 6

This soup is perfect for those cold winter nights when you want to relax with a comforting grilled cheese and tomato soup combo. The slow roasting of the tomatoes gives it tons of flavor.

- 1 (28-OUNCE) CAN PEELED WHOLE TOMATOES, DRAINED
- ¼ CUP OLIVE OIL
- 1 TEASPOON DRIED ITALIAN SEASONING
- ½ SMALL RED ONION, CHOPPED
- 2 CLOVES GARLIC, ROUGH CHOPPED
- ¼ CUP CHICKEN BROTH
- ½ CUP RICOTTA CHEESE
- ½ CUP HEAVY CREAM

Add the tomatoes, olive oil, herbs, vegetables, and broth to slow cooker.

Cover and cook on low for about 6 hours, until the vegetables are soft.

Use a blender to puree the soup and transfer it back to the slow cooker, or use an immersion blender directly in the slow cooker.

Just before serving, stir in the ricotta and heavy cream. Serve hot.

Cream of Broccoli Soup

SERVES 4 TO 6

If you add a pinch of baking soda while cooking this soup, you'll preserve the bright green color that makes broccoli so appetizing. While most soups are better the next day, broccoli soup is an exception, as the strong sulfurous aroma intensifies the longer it sits. Because of that, you shouldn't let this soup go to waste.

1 TABLESPOON BUTTER
½ MEDIUM ONION, DICED
2 SMALL CARROTS, DICED
1 POUND BROCCOLI FLORETS
2 CUPS CHICKEN BROTH
1 PINCH BAKING SODA
½ CUP WHOLE MILK OR HALF-AND-HALF
SALT AND PEPPER, TO TASTE

Grease the inside of the slow cooker with cooking spray, butter, or oil.

Melt the butter in the slow cooker, and add the onion, carrots, and broccoli. Toss the vegetables in the butter. Add the broth and baking soda. Cover and cook on low for about 5 hours.

Just before serving, stir in the milk or half-and-half, and season with salt and pepper. Serve hot.

Ham and White Bean Soup

SERVES 4

Loaded with creamy white beans and spicy ham, this aromatic soup is a great stand-alone meal. This soup heats up beautifully the next day and is even more full of flavor. It pairs wonderfully with a sandwich for lunch. You may use dried beans, but you'll need to soak them overnight or cook the soup for several more hours in the slow cooker.

2 TABLESPOONS OLIVE OIL, OPTIONAL
2 OUNCES SPICY ITALIAN HAM, CHOPPED
1 SMALL ONION, DICED
1 CLOVE GARLIC, MINCED
2 CELERY STALKS, DICED
1 SMALL CARROT, DICED
1 (14-OUNCE) CAN CRUSHED TOMATOES, DRAINED
1 (14-OUNCE) CAN WHITE BEANS, DRAINED AND RINSED
3 CUPS CHICKEN BROTH
SALT AND PEPPER, TO TASTE

Grease the inside of the slow cooker with cooking spray, butter, or oil.

For deep flavor, sauté the ham, onion, garlic, celery, and carrot in the olive oil in a medium skillet set over medium-high heat for about 5 minutes, until the ham is crisp and the vegetables are tender. Add the cooked ham and vegetables to the slow cooker. If you are pressed for time or prefer to skip the extra fat, you can add the ham and vegetables directly to the slow cooker without pre-cooking, and omit the butter.

Add the tomatoes, beans, and broth. Season with salt and pepper, cover, and cook on low for 8 to 9 hours. Serve hot.

Hearty Bean Soup

SERVES 6 TO 8

Dried beans taste better and are healthier for you, but they aren't as convenient as canned. Luckily, they are perfect for the slow cooker. You can use either in this recipe, and you can use any combination of beans you'd like. The more varieties you use, the more colorful and flavorful your soup will be.

2 CUPS MIXED DRIED BEANS, SOAKED OVERNIGHT
1 SMALL ONION, CHOPPED
1 SMALL CARROT, CHOPPED
2 CELERY STALKS, CHOPPED
1 (14-OUNCE) CAN DICED TOMATOES
1 SMOKED HAM HOCK
6 CUPS CHICKEN BROTH
1 TEASPOON DRIED THYME
1 BAY LEAF
SALT AND PEPPER, TO TASTE

Add all of the ingredients to the slow cooker.

Cover and cook on low for 8 to 10 hours until the ham is falling off the bone.

Remove the ham bone, strip off any meat, and add the meat back to the pot.

Remove the bay leaf, taste and adjust seasonings as needed, and serve hot.

Chicken and Wild Rice Soup

SERVES 4 TO 6

Moist and tender chunks of slow-cooked chicken pair wonderfully with the firmness of the wild rice in this soup. While there are a few steps to get this soup started, the end result is well worth the trouble and the wait. If you have cooked turkey on hand, you can use that instead of chicken; both are delicious.

2 TABLESPOONS BUTTER, OPTIONAL
1 SMALL ONION, CHOPPED
2 SMALL CARROTS, CHOPPED
1 POUND BUTTON MUSHROOMS, SLICED
6 CUPS CHICKEN BROTH
2 CUPS COOKED, SHREDDED CHICKEN
1 CUP WILD RICE, RINSED IN COLD WATER
1 TEASPOON DRIED THYME
1 TEASPOON DRIED SAGE
SALT AND PEPPER, TO TASTE
½ CUP HEAVY CREAM

Grease the inside of the slow cooker with cooking spray, butter, or oil.

For deep flavor, sauté the onion, carrots, and mushrooms in the butter in a medium skillet set over medium-high heat for about 5 minutes, until the vegetables begin to soften and the onion becomes translucent. Add the cooked vegetables to the slow cooker. If you are pressed for time or prefer to skip the extra fat, you can add the vegetables directly to the slow cooker without pre-cooking, and omit the butter.

Add the broth, chicken, rice, thyme, sage, salt, and pepper. Cover and cook on low for 5 hours.

Stir in the cream, taste and adjust seasonings as needed, and serve the soup hot.

Spicy Chicken Tortilla Soup

SERVES 4 TO 6

While this version has tender, shredded chicken, you can easily make a vegetarian dish by substituting 2 cups of cooked black beans for the chicken. You can make your own tortilla chips by cutting corn tortillas into strips and frying them in vegetable oil. For a super low-fuss meal, a bag of tortilla chips works great.

2 TABLESPOONS OLIVE OIL, OPTIONAL
1 SMALL RED BELL PEPPER, SEEDED AND DICED
1 SMALL GREEN BELL PEPPER, SEEDED AND DICED
1 SMALL YELLOW BELL PEPPER, SEEDED AND DICED
1 MEDIUM WHITE ONION, DICED
2 CLOVES GARLIC, CHOPPED
1 TABLESPOON CHILI POWDER
1 TABLESPOON CUMIN
1 (14-OUNCE) CAN DICED TOMATOES, DRAINED
3 CUPS CHICKEN BROTH
2 CUPS COOKED, SHREDDED CHICKEN
SALT AND PEPPER, TO TASTE
BROKEN TORTILLA CHIPS, SHREDDED CHEESE, AVOCADO,
   AND SOUR CREAM, FOR GARNISH

Grease the inside of the slow cooker with cooking spray, butter, or oil.

For deep flavor, sauté the bell peppers, onion, and garlic in the oil in a medium skillet set over medium-high heat for about 5 minutes, until the vegetables begin to soften and the onion becomes translucent. Stir in the chili powder and cumin and cook, stirring, for another minute. Add the cooked vegetables to the slow cooker. If you are pressed for time or prefer to skip the extra fat, you can add the vegetables and spices directly to the slow cooker without pre-cooking, and omit the oil.

Add the tomatoes, broth, chicken, salt, and pepper. Cover the pot and cook on low for 7 to 8 hours. Taste and adjust seasonings as needed.

To serve, ladle the hot soup into bowls and top with desired garnishes.

• Soups and Stews •

Summer Vegetable Soup

SERVES 6

You don't always think of soup in the summer, but if you have a lot of fresh produce left at season's end, the best way to use it up is in a pot of soup. Of course, you can enjoy this soup any time by using frozen vegetables; just be sure to thaw them before adding them to the slow cooker.

2 TABLESPOONS VEGETABLE OIL, OPTIONAL
1 SMALL ONION, CHOPPED
2 SMALL CELERY STALKS, CHOPPED
1 POUND NEW POTATOES, PEELED AND DICED
1 POUND GREEN BEANS, TRIMMED AND CUT INTO BITE-SIZED PIECES
1 CUP CORN KERNELS
4 CUPS CHICKEN OR VEGETABLE BROTH
CHOPPED GREEN ONIONS AND SLICED RADISHES, FOR GARNISH

Grease the inside of the slow cooker with cooking spray, butter, or oil.

For deep flavor, sauté the onion and celery in the oil in a medium skillet set over medium-high heat for about 5 minutes, until the onion becomes translucent. Add the cooked vegetables to the slow cooker. If you are pressed for time or prefer to skip the extra fat, you can add the vegetables directly to the slow cooker without pre-cooking, and omit the oil.

Add the potatoes, green beans, corn, and broth. Cover and cook on low for 6 to 7 hours until the vegetables are tender. Serve hot, garnished with green onions and radish slices.

[Handwritten note: ADD Chicken, ZUC, MUSH]

CHAPTER FOUR

American Favorites

CHAPTER FOUR

American Favorites

In this chapter, you'll find all your favorite American comfort foods, from meatloaf and pot roast to baby back ribs. Most of these dishes are also fairly simple and require few steps, which make them easy weeknight dinners. If you know that you have a stressful day ahead, plan one of these dinners and you'll have a comforting dish waiting for you when you walk in the door.

Old-Fashioned Beef Stew

SERVES 6 TO 8

This is the type of dish a slow cooker was made for. For variation, you can use different types of meat. A pork shoulder works well, as does lamb and even chicken. You can even customize the vegetables to your choosing.

4 OR 5 MEDIUM YUKON GOLD POTATOES, QUARTERED
2 MEDIUM CARROTS, CUT IN LARGE CHUNKS
2 SMALL ONIONS, QUARTERED
1 TEASPOON SALT, PLUS ADDITIONAL FOR SEASONING THE MEAT
½ TEASPOON PEPPER, PLUS ADDITIONAL FOR SEASONING THE MEAT
1 TEASPOON DRIED THYME
2 POUNDS BEEF CHUCK, TRIMMED AND CUT INTO 1-INCH PIECES
½ CUP FLOUR
1 TABLESPOON OLIVE OIL
1 CUP BEEF BROTH
1 CUP PEAS
1 CUP WHOLE CORN

Grease the inside of the slow cooker with cooking spray, butter, or oil.

Add the potatoes, carrots, onions, salt, pepper, and thyme to the slow cooker.

Season the meat with salt and pepper. Put the flour in a plastic freezer bag and add the meat. Shake until the pieces of meat are evenly coated with flour.

Heat the oil in a large skillet over medium-high heat. Add the beef and cook, turning it occasionally, until the meat is browned on all sides, about 6 to 8 minutes. Transfer the meat to the slow cooker. Add the broth to the skillet and bring to a boil, scraping up the browned bits from the bottom of the pan, then pour it into the slow cooker over the meat. Cover and cook on low for 8 to 10 hours until the meat is tender and the sauce has thickened.

Add the peas and corn and cook for an additional hour. Season with more salt and pepper, if desired, and serve.

Shredded Buffalo Chicken

SERVES 4 TO 6

This is perhaps one of the easiest slow cooker recipes you'll try. It produces tender, shredded, spicy buffalo chicken that you can use on sandwiches, quesadillas, pizzas, and more. Serve with blue cheese dressing for an authentic buffalo chicken taste.

½ CUP BUTTER, MELTED
5 LARGE SKINLESS CHICKEN BREASTS
½ CUP HOT SAUCE OF YOUR CHOICE
SALT, TO TASTE

Grease the inside of the slow cooker with cooking spray, butter, or oil.

Add the butter to the slow cooker. Add the chicken breasts, layering as you go with the hot sauce.

Cover and cook on low for 5 to 6 hours, turning the chicken breasts after about 2 hours.

When the chicken is done, remove it from the pot and shred it with two forks, discarding the bones. Add the chicken back to the pot and stir to coat it with the buttery buffalo sauce. Taste and add salt, if needed.

Serve warm.

Pulled-Pork Barbecue

SERVES 8

Barbecue is one of those things that everyone has a different opinion about. Some like a sweet sauce, while others claim that spicy is the only way to go. One thing all barbecue fans can agree on is that if the meat's not tender, it doesn't matter what kind of sauce it's cooked in. Tough meat just isn't worth the trouble. A slow braise in a slow cooker really tenderizes the flavorful pork in this dish.

1½ CUPS KETCHUP
1 MEDIUM ONION, CHOPPED
¼ CUP VEGETABLE OIL
2 TABLESPOONS RED WINE VINEGAR
½ CUP (PACKED) DARK BROWN SUGAR
¼ CUP SOY SAUCE
2 TABLESPOONS WORCESTERSHIRE SAUCE
1 TEASPOON GARLIC POWDER
3- TO 4-POUND BONELESS PORK SHOULDER, TRIMMED OF VISIBLE FAT

Grease the inside of the slow cooker with cooking spray, butter, or oil.

Combine the ketchup, onion, oil, vinegar, sugar, soy sauce, Worcestershire sauce, and garlic powder in a large plastic bag. Put the pork in the bag with the mixture, tossing to coat the entire piece. Refrigerate the pork for 6 to 8 hours, turning the bag once.

Alow the bag to come to room temperature, and pour the entire contents into the slow cooker. Cover and cook on low for 10 hours or until the pork is tender.

Remove the meat from the slow cooker and shred it with two forks. Add the meat back to the slow cooker and stir to coat the meat with the sauce. Serve hot directly from the slow cooker.

Old-Fashioned Meatloaf

SERVES 6

There are many meatloaf recipes out there, and everyone has their favorite. This is a traditional version with onion and bell pepper that uses cracker crumbs as the filler. It's easy to put together, and once it's in the slow cooker, you don't have to worry about it. Serve with mashed potatoes and gravy for a home-style experience you won't forget.

2 TABLESPOONS OLIVE OIL
1 MEDIUM ONION, CHOPPED
1 SMALL GREEN BELL PEPPER, SEEDED AND CHOPPED
1 TEASPOON DRIED SAGE
1½ POUNDS GROUND BEEF
1 CUP CRACKER CRUMBS
2 EGGS, BEATEN
1 CUP BEEF BROTH, DIVIDED
2 TABLESPOONS KETCHUP
1 TABLESPOON WORCESTERSHIRE SAUCE
1 TEASPOON SALT

Grease the inside of the slow cooker with cooking spray, butter, or oil.

Heat the oil in a large skillet over medium-high heat. Add the onion and bell pepper. Cook until tender and add the sage.

Transfer the mixture to a mixing bowl and add the beef, cracker crumbs, eggs, ½ cup of broth, ketchup, Worcestershire sauce, and salt. Mix by hand until well combined, but don't over mix.

Pat the meat into a loaf shape that will fit in the slow cooker. Add the remaining broth to the slow cooker followed by the meatloaf. Cover the pot and cook on high for 1 hour. Reduce the heat to low, and cook for an additional 4 to 6 hours, until an instant-read thermometer inserted in the center reads 165 degrees F.

Carefully transfer the meatloaf from the pot to a cutting board. Allow to rest for about 10 minutes. Slice and serve.

Barbecued Baby Back Ribs

SERVES 6

Cooking ribs in the slow cooker is easy because you don't have to be home all day while they cook. Fall-off-the-bone tender, these ribs have a lip-smacking sweet and spicy flavor that everyone loves. You can adjust the spices and seasonings in the sauce to tailor it to your personal preference.

4 POUNDS BABY BACK RIBS
2 CUPS KETCHUP
½ CUP APPLE CIDER
½ CUP (PACKED) BROWN SUGAR
¼ CUP DIJON MUSTARD
1 TABLESPOON WORCESTERSHIRE SAUCE
1 TABLESPOON HOT SAUCE
1 TEASPOON SALT

Grease the inside of the slow cooker with cooking spray, butter, or oil.

Cut the ribs to fit into the slow cooker and add them along with the rest of the ingredients. Cover and cook on low for 8 to 9 hours until the meat is tender and falling off the bone.

To serve, cut or pull the ribs apart and serve with the sauce on the side.

Pork Chops with Apples and Sauerkraut

SERVES 4

If you think of pork chops as being dry and tough, then you've never had them cooked in a slow cooker. Surprisingly melt-in-your-mouth tender, you'll never want to cook pork chops any other way.

¼ CUP BUTTER, MELTED
4 APPLES, PEELED, CORED, AND SLICED
¼ CUP DIJON MUSTARD
¼ CUP (PACKED) BROWN SUGAR
4 PORK CHOPS, CUT INTO 1-INCH PIECES
1 MEDIUM ONION, SLICED
1 POUND SAUERKRAUT, DRAINED AND RINSED
½ CUP APPLE CIDER

Grease the inside of the slow cooker with cooking spray, butter, or oil.

Pour the butter into the slow cooker, add the apple slices, and toss to coat. Stir the mustard and sugar together in a small bowl and add it to the apples. Add the pork chops, followed by the onion and sauerkraut. Pour the apple cider over the top. Cover and cook on low for 6 to 8 hours or until the pork is tender.

Serve the pork chops with the apples and sauerkraut.

Franks and Beans

SERVES 6

This is super easy to make in a slow cooker, and it makes a great dish for kids if you're having a sleepover or birthday party. Dried beans are called for in this recipe, but you can use canned and skip the overnight soaking if that's what you have on hand.

2 CUPS WHITE BEANS, SOAKED OVERNIGHT AND DRAINED
4 SLICES BACON, CUT INTO 1-INCH PIECES
4 CUPS VEGETABLE BROTH
1 MEDIUM ONION, CHOPPED
1 CLOVE GARLIC, MINCED
¼ CUP MOLASSES
¼ CUP YELLOW MUSTARD
2 TABLESPOONS BROWN SUGAR
PINCH OF GROUND GINGER
8 HOT DOGS, CUT INTO BITE-SIZED PIECES
½ TEASPOON SALT OR TO TASTE

Grease the inside of the slow cooker with cooking spray, butter, or oil.

Add the beans to the slow cooker.

Cook the bacon in a medium skillet until it's just short of crisp. Add the broth to the skillet and scrape up the brown bits from the bottom of the pan. Transfer the bacon and broth to the slow cooker. Stir in the onion, garlic, molasses, mustard, sugar, ginger, hot dogs, and salt. Cover and cook on low for 10 hours or until the beans are tender and the sauce is thickened. Serve hot.

Chicken Potpie

SERVES 6

While this dish doesn't have the flaky pastry top you associate with potpies, it does have a mashed potato topping that gets slightly crisp and is a delicious alternative. If you have leftover mashed potatoes, this is a great opportunity to use them up.

3 CUPS CHICKEN BROTH
3 TO 4 YUKON GOLD POTATOES, PEELED AND CUT INTO CUBES
2 CUPS BABY CARROTS
1 TEASPOON DRIED THYME
2 TABLESPOONS FLOUR
2 TABLESPOONS BUTTER, AT ROOM TEMPERATURE
3 CUPS COOKED AND SHREDDED OR CHOPPED CHICKEN
1 CUP PEAS
1 CUP CORN
2 CUPS PREPARED MASHED POTATOES

Grease the inside of the slow cooker with cooking spray, butter, or oil.

Add the broth to the slow cooker along with the potatoes, carrots, and thyme. Stir to combine, cover, and cook on high for 3 hours or until the potatoes are tender.

In a small bowl, combine the flour and butter to form a paste.

Add the butter mixture, chicken, peas, and corn to the slow cooker. Stir to combine. Spread the mashed potatoes on top and cook for 1 hour.

Serve hot from the pot.

Classic Pot Roast

SERVES 6

You can make a pot roast many ways, but there are none as simple as this classic style. Throw a big slab of meat into the slow cooker with some stock and vegetables and the end result is a mouthwatering, tender roast that is hard to beat. You can skip browning the roast if you're in a hurry, but you'll miss out on some flavor.

3 TABLESPOONS OLIVE OIL
3 TO 4 POUNDS CHUCK ROAST
SALT AND PEPPER, TO TASTE
1 CUP BABY CARROTS
2 POUNDS POTATOES, ANY TYPE, CUT INTO SMALL CHUNKS
1 ONION, SLICED
2 CUPS BEEF BROTH

Grease the inside of the slow cooker with cooking spray, butter, or oil.

Heat the oil in a large skillet. Season the roast with salt and pepper, and add it to the pan. Sear on all sides until well browned.

Place the vegetables in the bottom of the slow cooker. Pour the stock over them and add the roast. Cover and cook on low for 10 to 12 hours or until the roast is tender.

Transfer the roast from the slow cooker to a cutting board and let rest for 10 minutes. To serve, slice the roast thinly against the grain and serve with the vegetables alongside.

CHAPTER FIVE

International Dishes

CHAPTER FIVE

International Dishes

The slow cooker is a great tool for cooking many international dishes. The long cooking time also allows the flavors of exotic spices to fully permeate the dishes. No matter what your favorite cuisine, you are sure to find some favorite recipes you'll come back to again and again.

Tandoori Chicken

SERVES 4

For a more authentic flavor in this traditional Indian dish, you can toast the spices in a dry skillet. Simply add the spices to the skillet (you can add them all at once) and turn on the heat. Shake the pan and watch what you're doing as they can burn quickly. You'll know they are almost done when you start to smell the strong aromas coming from the skillet.

1 CUP PLAIN YOGURT
1 TABLESPOON LEMON JUICE
2 CLOVES GARLIC, CHOPPED
1 TEASPOON CORIANDER
1 TEASPOON PAPRIKA
1 TEASPOON SALT
½ TEASPOON CUMIN
½ TEASPOON GROUND CARDAMOM
2 TO 3 POUNDS CHICKEN, CUT INTO 8 PIECES

Grease the inside of the slow cooker with cooking spray, butter, or oil.

In a 1-gallon plastic bag, combine the yogurt, lemon juice, garlic, coriander, paprika, salt, cumin, and cardamom. Add the chicken and shake to coat the pieces well. Refrigerate for 8 hours or overnight.

Empty the plastic bag into the slow cooker, cover, and cook on low for 8 hours or until the chicken is cooked through.

Serve the chicken hot over rice.

• International Dishes •

Moroccan Chicken Tagine

SERVES 4

This is a stew-like dish that is richly seasoned and most often served with rice or couscous. This version is loaded with dried fruit and is a warmly spiced, sweet, and savory dish that you'll love. Use any variety of dried fruit; raisins or even dried mangoes will work well here.

¼ CUP OLIVE OIL, OPTIONAL
½ TEASPOON SALT, PLUS ADDITIONAL FOR SEASONING THE MEAT
½ TEASPOON PEPPER, PLUS ADDITIONAL FOR SEASONING THE MEAT
8 SKINLESS, BONELESS CHICKEN THIGHS
2 CUPS CHICKEN BROTH
1 MEDIUM ONION, CHOPPED
½ CUP DRIED APRICOTS, CHOPPED
½ CUP DRIED PLUMS
JUICE AND ZEST OF 1 ORANGE
2 CLOVES GARLIC, MINCED
1 TABLESPOON BROWN SUGAR
1 TEASPOON GROUND TURMERIC
½ TEASPOON GROUND CUMIN
½ TEASPOON GROUND GINGER
⅛ TEASPOON CAYENNE
2 TABLESPOONS COLD WATER MIXED WITH 2 TABLESPOONS CORNSTARCH

Grease the inside of the slow cooker with cooking spray, butter, or oil.

Heat the oil in a large skillet. Season the chicken with salt and pepper. Cook the chicken, turning once, until it is browned on both sides. Transfer the chicken to the slow cooker.

Add the broth, onion, dried fruit, orange zest and juice, garlic, sugar, turmeric, cumin, ginger, cayenne, and the remaining ½ teaspoon of salt and ½ teaspoon of pepper. Cover and cook on high for about 5 hours or until the chicken is tender.

Add the cornstarch mixture, stir, and continue to cook, covered, for about 30 minutes until the sauce thickens.

Serve hot over rice or couscous.

Miso Chicken with Broccoli

SERVES 4

This is a delicious and super healthful dish that requires very little preparation. You can easily throw everything in the slow cooker before you leave for work in the morning and have a fully cooked meal when you get home. If you like your broccoli a little crisper, simply leave it out, and when you're ready to eat, add it to the pot and cook it for about fifteen minutes.

2 CUPS CHICKEN BROTH
¼ CUP WHITE MISO PASTE
1 CLOVE GARLIC, SMASHED
2 QUARTER-SIZED SLICES PEELED FRESH GINGER
½ TEASPOON SALT
4 BONELESS, SKINLESS CHICKEN BREAST HALVES
1 POUND BROCCOLI FLORETS

Grease the inside of the slow cooker with cooking spray, butter, or oil.

Combine the chicken broth, miso, garlic, ginger, and salt in the slow cooker. Add the chicken and broccoli and toss to coat. Cover and cook on low for 6 to 8 hours or until the chicken is tender and falling apart.

Serve with rice or udon noodles for an authentic Japanese meal.

North African Beef Stew

SERVES 6

As this dish cooks, it will fill your home with the pleasant fragrance of the spices found in traditional African markets. The dish itself is filled with hearty chunks of tender beef, soft and plump dried fruit, and garbanzo beans that pair wonderfully with couscous or rice.

1 TEASPOON SALT, PLUS ADDITIONAL FOR SEASONING THE MEAT
3 POUNDS BEEF CHUCK ROAST, CUT INTO BITE-SIZED PIECES
2 TABLESPOONS OLIVE OIL
1 MEDIUM ONION, CHOPPED
2 LARGE CARROTS, CHOPPED
2 CLOVES GARLIC, CHOPPED
2 TEASPOONS PAPRIKA
1 TEASPOON CUMIN
½ TEASPOON CINNAMON
3 CUPS BEEF BROTH
2 CUPS GARBANZO BEANS
1 CUP DRIED APRICOTS, CHOPPED
½ CUP GOLDEN RAISINS
2 TABLESPOONS CORNSTARCH MIXED WITH 2 TABLESPOONS COLD WATER

Grease the inside of the slow cooker with cooking spray, butter, or oil.

Season the beef with salt. In a large skillet set over medium-high heat, sauté the beef in the olive oil until it is browned on all sides. Transfer the beef to the slow cooker. Add the onion, carrots, and garlic to the skillet and cook until the onion is soft, about 3 minutes. Add the paprika, cumin, and cinnamon and cook 1 minute more. Transfer the vegetable mixture to the slow cooker. Stir in the broth, beans, dried apricots, raisins, and the remaining 1 teaspoon of salt. Cover and cook for 10 hours on low or until the meat is tender and falling apart.

Add the cornstarch mixture, stir, and continue to cook, covered, for about 30 minutes until the sauce thickens.

Serve hot over rice or couscous.

Osso Bucco

SERVES 4

A traditional Italian veal dish, osso bucco is usually served with risotto. Gremolata, a chopped mixture of parsley, lemon, and garlic, is usually sprinkled on top, but here it's simply added to the pot for a unique depth of flavor. When cooked all day, the veal becomes succulent and mouthwatering, and practically melts in your mouth.

4 (2-INCH) VEAL SHANKS
½ TEASPOON SALT, PLUS ADDITIONAL FOR SEASONING THE MEAT
¼ TEASPOON PEPPER, PLUS ADDITIONAL FOR SEASONING THE MEAT
½ CUP FLOUR
2 TABLESPOONS OLIVE OIL
1 MEDIUM ONION, CHOPPED
2 CARROTS, CHOPPED
¼ CUP TOMATO PASTE
½ CUP DRY WHITE WINE
1 CUP CHICKEN BROTH
½ CUP BEEF BROTH
2 CLOVES GARLIC, MINCED
ZEST OF 1 LEMON
½ CUP FINELY CHOPPED PARSLEY

Grease the inside of the slow cooker with cooking spray, butter, or oil.

Season the veal with salt and pepper, and coat with the flour.

Heat the oil in a large skillet. Add the veal and cook until browned on all sides. Add the onion and carrots, and cook until soft, about 3 minutes.

Transfer the veal and sautéed vegetables to the slow cooker. Add the tomato paste, wine, chicken broth, beef broth, garlic, lemon zest, parsley, and the remaining ½ teaspoon of salt and ¼ teaspoon of pepper. Cover and cook for 6 to 8 hours on low until the veal is tender.

Serve hot with risotto or pasta.

• International Dishes •

Curried Coconut Chicken with Basil

SERVES 4

With the combination of spicy curry powder and sweet coconut milk, this dish is a medley of contrasting flavors. You can serve this with a variety of condiments, including Indian chutney, toasted coconut, hard-boiled egg, bacon, or toasted peanuts.

4 TABLESPOONS BUTTER, OPTIONAL
1 MEDIUM ONION, CHOPPED
8 BONELESS, SKINLESS CHICKEN THIGHS
1 TEASPOON SALT, PLUS ADDITIONAL FOR SEASONING THE CHICKEN
1 TEASPOON GARAM MASALA
1 TEASPOON GINGER, GRATED
1 LARGE APPLE, CORED, PEELED, AND CHOPPED
½ CUP FLOUR
2 CUPS CHICKEN BROTH
1 TEASPOON CURRY POWDER
1 CUP COCONUT MILK
¼ CUP FRESHLY SLICED BASIL

Grease the inside of the slow cooker with cooking spray, butter, or oil.

For the best flavor, sauté the onion in the butter until tender. Season the chicken with salt and add it to the onion in the skillet. Cook the chicken, turning once, until it is browned on both sides, and then transfer the chicken and onion to the slow cooker along with the remaining ingredients except for the basil. If you are pressed for time, simply omit the butter and add all of the ingredients, except for the basil, to the slow cooker at once.

Cover and cook for 6 to 8 hours on low or until the chicken is tender.

Serve hot, garnished with the basil.

Kielbasa and Sauerkraut

SERVES 4

This super easy dish is perfect for a cold winter day, or anytime you're looking for a slow cooker dish that you don't have to prep. With so few ingredients, you simply throw everything in the pot and cover. A few hours later, you'll have a hearty, flavorful meal that's ready when you are.

1 POUND KIELBASA OR SMOKED SAUSAGE OF YOUR CHOICE, CUT INTO ½-INCH PIECES
2 CUPS CHICKEN BROTH
2 CUPS SAUERKRAUT, DRAINED

Grease the inside of the slow cooker with cooking spray, butter, or oil.

Combine all the ingredients in the slow cooker. Cover and cook on low for 4 to 5 hours or until the sausage is heated through.

Serve the sausage with the sauerkraut.

• International Dishes •

Veal Paprikash

SERVES 4

For the best results when making this dish, be sure that the paprika is fresh. Serve this traditional dish with dumplings or, for the most authentic experience, with spaetzle.

5 SLICES BACON, CHOPPED
2 POUNDS VEAL SHANK, CUT INTO BITE-SIZED PIECES
1 TEASPOON SALT, PLUS ADDITIONAL FOR SEASONING THE MEAT
½ TEASPOON PEPPER, PLUS ADDITIONAL FOR SEASONING THE MEAT
½ CUP FLOUR
1 MEDIUM ONION, CHOPPED
1 LARGE GREEN BELL PEPPER, SEEDED AND CHOPPED
1 LARGE RED BELL PEPPER, SEEDED AND CHOPPED
1 (15-OUNCE) CAN CRUSHED TOMATOES
1 CUP CHICKEN BROTH
1 CUP BEEF BROTH
2 TABLESPOONS SWEET PAPRIKA
1 TEASPOON DRIED THYME
¼ TEASPOON HOT PAPRIKA
1 BAY LEAF
1 CUP SOUR CREAM, AT ROOM TEMPERATURE

Grease the inside of the slow cooker with cooking spray, butter, or oil.

Cook the bacon in a large skillet until crisp. Add it to the slow cooker. Season the veal with salt and pepper, and coat it with the flour. Add it to the pan you used for the bacon, and cook until browned on all sides. Transfer the meat to the slow cooker.

Add the onions and peppers to the skillet and cook until soft, about 5 minutes. Transfer to the slow cooker along with the tomatoes, chicken broth, beef broth, sweet paprika, thyme, hot paprika, bay leaf, and the remaining teaspoon of salt and ½ teaspoon of pepper.

Cover and cook on high for 5 to 6 hours. Remove the bay leaf, stir in the sour cream, and serve.

Mexican-Style Pork

SERVES 4

This recipe has a smoky and spicy flavor that is perfect for tacos or even served over Mexican-style rice. Cheese, extra salsa, and avocado are wonderful garnishes for this tender and delicious dish.

2 TABLESPOONS OLIVE OIL, OPTIONAL
½ CUP ONION, CHOPPED
2 CLOVES GARLIC, MINCED
2 POUNDS BONELESS PORK SHOULDER, CUT INTO BITE-SIZED PIECES
1 TEASPOON SALT, PLUS ADDITIONAL FOR SEASONING THE MEAT
2 CUPS WHOLE CORN
1 CUP PREPARED SALSA
½ CUP BEEF BROTH
1 TEASPOON GROUND CUMIN
½ TEASPOON CHILI POWDER

Grease the inside of the slow cooker with cooking spray, butter, or oil.

For deep flavor, sauté the onion and garlic in the olive oil in a skillet set over medium-high heat for about 5 minutes until tender. Transfer the mixture to the slow cooker. Season the pork with salt and cook it in the same skillet, turning a few times, until browned on all sides, about 6 minutes, and then transfer it to the slow cooker. If you prefer, simply omit the olive oil and add the onion, garlic, and pork directly to the slow cooker without pre-cooking.

Add the corn, salsa, broth, cumin, chili powder, and remaining 1 teaspoon of salt to the slow cooker. Cover and cook on low for 8 hours until the pork is tender. Serve with tortillas or rice.

• International Dishes •

Braised Asian Beef

SERVES 6

This dish is easy and delicious. Tender beef braised in Asian flavors is better than anything you'll get at a restaurant. Serve this with white rice for an authentic dish, although fried rice is great, too.

2 POUNDS CHUCK ROAST
SALT AND PEPPER, TO TASTE
2 TABLESPOONS VEGETABLE OIL
2 CUPS BEEF BROTH
½ CUP ORANGE JUICE
½ CUP SOY SAUCE
1 TEASPOON GROUND GINGER
½ TEASPOON RED PEPPER FLAKES
CHOPPED GREEN ONIONS AND SESAME SEEDS, FOR GARNISH

Grease the inside of the slow cooker with cooking spray, butter, or oil.

Season the roast with salt and pepper.

Heat the oil in a large skillet and cook the roast until it is browned on all sides, about 6 minutes. Transfer the roast to the slow cooker. Add the broth, orange juice, soy sauce, ginger, and red pepper flakes.

Cover and cook on low for 10 hours until the beef is tender.

Remove the roast from the slow cooker and let rest for 10 minutes. Slice thinly against the grain and serve garnished with green onions and sesame seeds.

Mediterranean Lamb

SERVES 4

Traditional Mediterranean cuisine relies heavily on the flavors of olive oil, mint, and garlic, and this dish is no exception. This is a one-pot meal that produces mouthwatering and tender chunks of lamb alongside green beans and garlic-flavored potatoes.

1 TEASPOON SALT, PLUS ADDITIONAL FOR SEASONING THE MEAT
½ TEASPOON PEPPER, PLUS ADDITIONAL FOR SEASONING THE MEAT
1½ POUNDS LAMB SHOULDER, CUT INTO BITE-SIZED PIECES
¼ CUP OLIVE OIL, DIVIDED
1½ POUNDS SMALL POTATOES, HALVED
½ POUND FRESH GREEN BEANS, TRIMMED
4 CLOVES GARLIC, MINCED
1 MEDIUM ONION, CHOPPED
½ CUP CHICKEN BROTH
2 TABLESPOONS DRY WHITE WINE
2 TABLESPOONS TOMATO PASTE
2 TABLESPOONS FRESH MINT, CHOPPED

Grease the inside of the slow cooker with cooking spray, butter, or oil.

Season the lamb with salt and pepper. Heat 2 tablespoons of oil in a large skillet set over medium-high heat and cook the lamb, stirring, until it is browned on all sides.

Place the the potatoes, green beans, garlic, and the remaining 2 tablespoons of olive oil, 1 teaspoon of salt, and ½ teaspoon of pepper in the slow cooker. Transfer the lamb from the skillet to the slow cooker on top of the vegetables.

Add the onion, chicken broth, wine, tomato paste, and mint to the slow cooker. Cover and cook on low for 8 to 10 hours or until the lamb is tender and the potatoes can be easily pierced with a fork.

Serve the lamb and vegetables with a bit of the sauce spooned over the top.

CHAPTER SIX

Fish and Seafood

CHAPTER SIX

Fish and Seafood

While fish and shellfish don't benefit from the long cooking times associated with a slow cooker, this doesn't mean you can't cook them. You just have to add them near the end of the cooking time and keep an eye on them to make sure they don't overcook. In general, meatier fish will work best in the cooker, but any type will do as long as it's not left in too long. Even a short cooking time will allow delicate fish filets and seafood to absorb the flavors in the slow cooker. While fish isn't something you're going to put in the pot before you leave for work, it's not that much trouble to add the seafood when you arrive home, so you can still end up with delicious and flavorful results.

Some types of fish work well in a slow cooker. Halibut, salmon, and tuna are all meaty cuts that can take a long cooking time. Lighter fish like tilapia, flounder, or other mild white fish tend to fall apart after only a few minutes.

Clams, mussels, and shellfish work well but will become tough and rubbery if overcooked, so be extremely careful and watch your cooking times.

Bouillabaisse

SERVES 6

Bouillabaisse is a classic dish from the Mediterranean region of France. There are many variations, but the basic version includes two things: an aromatic fish stock made with vegetables and herbs, and fish. The dish originated as a fisherman's stew that was composed of the catch of the day. For that reason, what kind of fish you use is your choice, although your options may be a little bit more limited using the slow cooker.

2 TABLESPOONS OLIVE OIL, OPTIONAL

3 LARGE LEEKS, WHITE AND LIGHT GREEN PARTS, CHOPPED

3 CLOVES GARLIC, CHOPPED

1 FENNEL BULB, TRIMMED AND COARSELY CHOPPED

1 (28-OUNCE) CAN CRUSHED TOMATOES WITH JUICE

½ CUP WHITE WINE

ZEST OF 1 ORANGE

1 TEASPOON DRIED THYME

1 TEASPOON SAFFRON, CRUMBLED

1 TEASPOON SALT

½ TEASPOON PEPPER

2 CUPS CLAM JUICE

1 CUP CHICKEN OR FISH BROTH

½ POUND LITTLENECK CLAMS

½ POUND MUSSELS

2 POUNDS THICK HALIBUT FILETS, CUT INTO CHUNKS

½ CUP FRESH PARSLEY, CHOPPED, FOR GARNISH

Grease the inside of the slow cooker with cooking spray, butter, or oil.

Heat the olive oil in a large skillet set over medium-high heat. Add the leeks, garlic, and fennel and cook, stirring ocassionally, until soft, about 5 minutes. Add the tomatoes, wine, zest, thyme, saffron, salt, and pepper. Bring to a boil and then reduce the heat to medium-low and simmer for about 10 minutes. Transfer the mixture to the slow cooker. Stir in the clam juice and broth, cover, and cook on low for 6 hours.

continued ▶

Bouillabasse *continued* ▶

Remove the lid and add the clams and mussels and then the fish on top. Replace the cover and cook another 30 to 45 minutes or until the fish is cooked through and flakes easily with a fork and the clam and mussel shells have opened. Be careful not to cook it for too long.

Discard any clams or mussels that are not open. Serve immediately, garnished with the chopped parsley.

Poached Tuna

SERVES 4 TO 6

When you buy tuna at the grocery store in cans and pouches, you get white, flavorless tuna that will make an acceptable tuna salad in a pinch, but there is another way. Raw tuna fillets cooked in a slow cooker with some olive oil produce a succulent, tender tuna that melts in your mouth. This is the most basic recipe and will work well in almost any dish containing tuna, but feel free to experiment with other flavorings. Garlic, lemon zest, or red pepper flakes are great options.

3 POUNDS TUNA FILLETS
OLIVE OIL TO COVER, ABOUT 2 CUPS
1 TEASPOON SALT

Grease the inside of the slow cooker with cooking spray, butter, or oil.

Put the tuna in the slow cooker and cover it with the olive oil. Add the salt, cover, and cook on low for 3 to 4 hours or until the tuna is white and tender.

Lemon and Garlic Halibut

SERVES 4

Halibut is a meaty white fish that absorbs flavors beautifully and is one of the best types of fish for the slow cooker. This dish is easy to prepare and makes for a great dinner when you're expecting company and you'll be at home for four or five hours to make the butter sauce before adding the fish. You can serve this with some mashed potatoes and a bottle of white wine for a dish that's easy, impressive, and delicious.

½ CUP BUTTER
¼ CUP OLIVE OIL
6 CLOVES GARLIC, MINCED
JUICE OF 2 LEMONS
ZEST OF 1 LEMON
¼ CUP FRESH CHIVES, CHOPPED
¾ TEASPOON SALT
½ TEASPOON SWEET PAPRIKA
4 THICK-CUT HALIBUT FILLETS
½ CUP FINELY CHOPPED FRESH PARSLEY, FOR GARNISH

Grease the inside of the slow cooker with cooking spray, butter, or oil.

Add the butter, oil, garlic, lemon juice, zest, chives, salt, and paprika to the slow cooker. Cover and cook on low for about 4 hours.

Add the halibut fillets to the slow cooker, cutting them to fit, if needed. Spoon the sauce lightly over the fish. Cover and cook for about 40 minutes until the fish is opaque and cooked through.

Serve garnished with the chopped parsley and drizzled with more sauce.

Sweet Miso-Glazed Cod

SERVES 4 TO 6

This is a surprisingly simple dish that produces the most delicious results. Black cod works well in this dish, but it can be hard to find. If you can't get your hands on black cod, then halibut, sea bass, or even salmon will work well here.

1 CUP WATER
½ CUP WHITE MISO PASTE
¼ CUP MIRIN
¼ CUP (PACKED) LIGHT BROWN SUGAR
1 TEASPOON RICE VINEGAR
2 POUNDS BLACK COD
SALT, TO TASTE
5 GREEN ONIONS, CHOPPED
¼ CUP SESAME SEEDS, TOASTED, FOR GARNISH

Grease the inside of the slow cooker with cooking spray, butter, or oil.

Combine the water, miso paste, mirin, brown sugar, and vinegar in the slow cooker. Cover and cook on low for 4 hours.

Add the fish to the slow cooker, cover, and cook for an additional 30 to 40 minutes or until the fish is tender. Transfer the fish from the slow cooker to a plate or cutting board and tent with foil to keep warm.

Transfer the remaining sauce to a small saucepan on the stove and bring to a boil. Cook for about 15 to 20 minutes until the sauce thickens and reduces by half. It should look syrupy. Taste and add salt if needed. Stir in the green onions.

Serve the fish with steamed white rice. Drizzle with the sauce, and sprinkle the toasted sesame seeds on top. Serve any extra sauce on the side.

Poached Salmon Cakes with White Wine Butter Sauce

SERVES 6

Salmon or other fish cakes are typically pan-fried for a crisp texture, but you may be surprised by this easy poached version. While not as crispy as a traditional salmon cake, this method of cooking leaves you with a super flavorful and tender cake that's delicious as an appetizer or as a meal on its own.

½ CUP BUTTER
1 TEASPOON OLD BAY SEASONING
2 CLOVES GARLIC, MINCED
2 CUPS WHITE WINE
4 CUPS COOKED SALMON, FLAKED WITH A FORK
6 OUNCES MARINATED ARTICHOKE HEARTS, DRAINED AND CHOPPED
1 CUP FRESH BREAD CRUMBS
½ CUP FRESHLY GRATED PARMESAN
1 EGG, BEATEN

Grease the inside of the slow cooker with cooking spray, butter, or oil.

Add the butter, Old Bay, garlic, and wine to the slow cooker. Cover and cook on low for 4 hours.

After you get the sauce started, place the rest of the ingredients in a large bowl, and mix to combine. Form the mixture into a dozen 2-inch patties and refrigerate.

Once the sauce has cooked, add the salmon cakes and cover with the sauce.

Cover and cook for 1 hour. The cakes will be tender when done.

Using a spatula or slotted spoon, carefully remove the cakes from the slow cooker.

Strain the remaining sauce and put it in a small saucepan. Bring to a boil and cook for 10 to 15 minutes or until it has reduced by about half and become a glaze.

Drizzle the cakes with the sauce, and serve the remaining sauce on the side.

Sea Bass with Spicy Crusted Potatoes

SERVES 6

Thinly sliced potatoes that have been seasoned with Creole spices envelop sea bass that has a delicately flavored lemon butter sauce. While the type of fish in most seafood dishes is interchangeable, you don't want to substitute the sea bass here. Sea bass has a different structure than other types of fish. If you insist on substituting, proceed with caution.

¼ CUP BUTTER, MELTED
JUICE AND ZEST OF 1 LEMON
2 CLOVES GARLIC, MINCED
3 TABLESPOONS OLIVE OIL, DIVIDED
1 TEASPOON SALT, DIVIDED
2 POUNDS SEA BASS FILLETS
5 OR 6 MEDIUM YUKON GOLD POTATOES, SLICED ABOUT ¼-INCH THICK
2 TABLESPOONS OLD BAY SEASONING

Grease the inside of the slow cooker with cooking spray, butter, or oil.

Combine the butter, lemon juice, zest, garlic, 2 tablespoons of olive oil, and ½ teaspoon of salt in a small bowl. Brush the fish fillets with the butter sauce and set aside.

In a large mixing bowl, combine the potatoes with the remaining tablespoon of olive oil, the Old Bay, and the remaining ½ teaspoon of salt.

Add half of the butter sauce to the slow cooker followed by half of the potatoes. Place the fish on top of the potatoes, cover with the remaining sauce, and top with the remaining potatoes.

Cover and cook on high for about 1½ hours until the potatoes start to brown and the sea bass is cooked through and opaque looking.

Remove the cover and cook for another 20 minutes.

Serve immediately.

Green Curried Shrimp

SERVES 4

This Thai dish is a combination of sweet, spicy, and fragrant. Some ingredients can be difficult to find at your regular grocery store; you may have to go to an Asian grocer. If you're not a fan of shrimp, firm tofu works equally as well in this dish, and you can add it in the beginning of the cook time for even easier preparation. Serve with brown jasmine rice for a hassle-free and healthful weeknight meal.

1 TABLESPOON VEGETABLE OIL, OPTIONAL
1 MEDIUM ONION, COARSELY CHOPPED
3 CLOVES GARLIC, MINCED
1 TABLESPOON FRESH GINGER, MINCED
1 (14-OUNCE) CAN COCONUT MILK
1 (10-INCH) STALK LEMONGRASS, ROOT END TRIMMED OFF AND TOUGH OUTER LEAVES REMOVED, CUT INTO 1-INCH PIECES
1 TABLESPOON THAI GREEN CURRY PASTE
1 TABLESPOON THAI FISH SAUCE (OR 1 TABLESPOON SOY SAUCE)
ZEST OF 1 SMALL LIME
1 TABLESPOON LIME JUICE
1 THAI CHILI PEPPER, SEEDED AND DICED
1½ POUNDS PEELED AND DEVEINED SHRIMP
½ CUP CHOPPED CILANTRO, FOR GARNISH
4 LIME WEDGES, FOR GARNISH

Grease the inside of the slow cooker with cooking spray, butter, or oil.

For deep flavor, sauté the onion, garlic, and ginger in the oil in a medium skillet set over medium-high heat for about 5 minutes, or until the onion is soft and translucent. Transfer the mixture to the slow cooker. If you are pressed for time, simply add the onion, garlic, and ginger to the slow cooker without pre-cooking, and omit the vegetable oil.

Add the coconut milk, lemongrass, curry paste, fish sauce, lime zest and juice, and chili. Cover and cook on low for about 4 hours.

continued ▶

Green Curried Shrimp *continued* ▶

Add the shrimp to the slow cooker and continue to cook, covered, for 5 to 10 minutes more until the shrimp are pink, being extra careful not to overcook.

Remove and discard the lemongrass pieces. Serve the shrimp garnished with the fresh cilantro and lime wedges over steamed jasmine rice.

CHAPTER SEVEN

Casseroles

CHAPTER SEVEN

Casseroles

For many people, slow cookers were made for casseroles, and it's no wonder. Nothing is quite as easy as layering pasta, rice, or other starches with meat, cheese, and vegetables, and coming home to a delicious comforting meal.

You'll find casseroles ranging from classics such as lasagna or tuna and noodles to more exotic dishes for those who aren't afraid to try something new. If you're looking for inspiration on what types of casseroles you can cook in a slow cooker, think about your favorites. You'll have a hard time finding a casserole that doesn't work perfectly in a slow cooker.

Tuna Noodle Casserole

SERVES 6 TO 8

This version of a classic is made with a homemade cream sauce and has flavorful mushrooms sautéed in butter throughout. As for the tuna, those water-packed versions just can't compare to a good oil-packed variety. Found jarred in gourmet markets, it is usually more expensive, but once you try it, you'll know it's worth the trouble.

8 OUNCES DRIED EGG NOODLES, COOKED AL DENTE ACCORDING TO PACKAGE DIRECTIONS
2 (6-OUNCE) JARS OIL-PACKED TUNA, DRAINED
¼ CUP BUTTER
1 SMALL ONION, CHOPPED
½ POUND BUTTON MUSHROOMS, SLICED
2 CELERY STALKS, CHOPPED
¼ CUP FLOUR
3 CUPS MILK
SALT AND PEPPER, TO TASTE
3 TO 4 DROPS HOT SAUCE

Grease the inside of the slow cooker with cooking spray, butter, or oil.

Add the noodles and tuna to the slow cooker, and stir to combine well.

Melt the butter in a medium saucepan set over medium-high heat. Add the onion, mushrooms, and celery and cook until the onion is soft and the mushrooms are starting to brown. Add the flour and continue to cook for 3 minutes until smooth and bubbly.

Slowly add the milk while constantly whisking. Season with salt and pepper and add the hot sauce. Bring to a boil, making sure to stir continuously.

Pour the milk mixture over the tuna and noodles in the slow cooker. Cover and cook on low for 4 to 5 hours.

Serve immediately.

• Casseroles •

Classic Lasagna Bolognese

SERVES 8

There are two ways to approach this recipe. You can make your own Bolognese sauce following the recipe below, or you can use a store-bought sauce and simmer it with some ground meat. You don't have to use no-boil noodles; regular lasagna noodles will work fine as long as they are covered with enough sauce. This lasagna recipe uses béchamel sauce instead of ricotta cheese.

FOR THE BOLOGNESE SAUCE:
2 TABLESPOONS OLIVE OIL
1 LARGE ONION, CHOPPED
2 LARGE CARROTS, CHOPPED
2 CELERY STALKS, CHOPPED
1 CLOVE GARLIC, MINCED
1 POUND LEAN GROUND BEEF
½ POUND GROUND VEAL
½ POUND GROUND PORK
PINCH OF NUTMEG
PINCH OF CINNAMON
SALT AND PEPPER, TO TASTE
1 CUP WHOLE MILK
3 (32-OUNCE) CANS OF CRUSHED TOMATOES
1 CUP DRY WHITE WINE

FOR THE LASAGNA:
4 TABLESPOONS BUTTER
¼ CUP FLOUR
1½ CUPS CHICKEN BROTH
1½ CUPS MILK
2 CUPS FRESHLY GRATED PARMESAN CHEESE, DIVIDED
1 (9-OUNCE) BOX LASAGNA NOODLES
1 POUND FRESH MOZZARELLA, SLICED

continued ▶

Bouillabasse *continued* ▶

To make the Bolognese sauce:

Grease the inside of the slow cooker with cooking spray, butter, or oil.

Heat the oil in a large skillet over medium-high heat. Add the onion, carrots, celery, and garlic. Cook for about 4 minutes or until vegetables are fragrant and tender. Add the ground meats and cook, stirring, until the meat is no longer pink.

Drain any fat from the pan. Add the nutmeg, cinnamon, salt, and pepper. Stir in the milk and bring to a boil. Cook until the liquid evaporates. Add the contents of the pan to the slow cooker along with the tomatoes and wine. Stir, cover, and cook on high for about 6 hours.

Sauce can be used immediately or refrigerated for about a week.

To make the lasagna:

Grease the inside of the slow cooker with cooking spray, butter, or oil.

Melt the butter in a saucepan over medium heat. Add the flour while stirring, and cook for 3 minutes until smooth and bubbly. Add the broth and milk, stirring continuously. Bring the mixture to a boil. Turn off heat, and stir in half of the Parmesan cheese.

Spoon some of the Bolognese sauce into the bottom of the slow cooker. Top with a layer of noodles, breaking them to fit if necessary. Add a layer of the white sauce, followed by mozzarella. Continue layering in this order until you have no more ingredients or the pot is three-quarters full. Be sure that you finish with a layer of the Bolognese sauce.

Sprinkle the rest of the Parmesan on top. Cover and cook on low for 4 to 5 hours or until bubbly. Remove the lid and continue cooking for 45 minutes to 1 hour.

Before serving, turn off the slow cooker and allow the lasagna to rest for 15 minutes. Slice into 8 pieces and serve hot.

Salmon, Artichoke, and Noodle Casserole

SERVES 8

This casserole is an upscale version of the tuna and noodle casserole you often see at potlucks and family gatherings. Tender chunks of salmon are interspersed throughout a creamy dill sauce and egg noodles. The artichokes add an additional depth of savory flavor that serves the dish well. You can customize it however you'd like by using noodles of your desired thickness, and you can even substitute shrimp.

8 OUNCES DRIED EGG NOODLES, COOKED AL DENTE ACCORDING TO PACKAGE DIRECTIONS
1 POUND COOKED SALMON, FLAKED
1 POUND FROZEN ARTICHOKE HEARTS, THAWED, DRAINED, AND CHOPPED
4 TABLESPOONS BUTTER
1 SMALL ONION, CHOPPED
3 TABLESPOONS FLOUR
3 CUPS MILK
¼ CUP CHOPPED FRESH DILL
SALT AND PEPPER, TO TASTE
½ CUP FRESH BREAD CRUMBS OR CRUSHED CRACKERS

Grease the inside of the slow cooker with cooking spray, butter, or oil.

Add the noodles, salmon, and artichoke hearts to the slow cooker. Stir to combine.

In a medium saucepan, melt the butter over medium heat and add the onion. Cook until tender, about 3 minutes. Add the flour and stir. Slowly add the milk and bring to a boil while stirring continuously. Boil for 1 minute, remove from heat, and stir in the dill.

Pour the milk mixture over the salmon and noodles and stir. Season with salt and pepper.

Cover and cook on low for 4 to 5 hours. Remove the lid, sprinkle the bread crumbs or crackers over the top, and cook, uncovered, for another 30 minutes.

Serve immediately.

Chicken and Mushroom Casserole

SERVES 8

If you've ever had a bland and boring chicken and rice casserole, then you'll greatly appreciate this dish. The chicken is cooked to tender perfection, while the casserole itself gets lots of flavor from sautéed mushrooms, dried fruit, and Marsala wine.

½ CUP BUTTER
1 MEDIUM ONION, CHOPPED
1 POUND MIXED MUSHROOMS SUCH AS CREMINI, SHIITAKE, AND OYSTER
1 TEASPOON DRIED THYME
SALT AND PEPPER, TO TASTE
¼ CUP MARSALA WINE
ZEST OF 1 LEMON
½ CUP DRIED APRICOTS, CHOPPED
3 CUPS COOKED CHICKEN, SHREDDED OR CHOPPED INTO BITE-SIZED PIECES
4 CUPS COOKED WILD RICE
2 CUPS CHICKEN BROTH

Grease the inside of the slow cooker with cooking spray, butter, or oil.

Heat a large skillet over medium-high heat and add the butter. When the butter is melted, add the onion, mushrooms, and thyme. Season with salt and pepper and sauté until the onion is soft and the mushrooms turn golden brown. Add the Marsala to the pan and remove from the heat.

Transfer the mushroom mixture to the slow cooker along with all of the remaining ingredients. Stir to combine thoroughly. Cover and cook for 2 to 3 hours or until the casserole is cooked through.

Remove the lid and cook until all of the liquid is absorbed, about 45 minutes.

Serve immediately.

CHAPTER EIGHT

Sides and Starters

CHAPTER EIGHT

Sides and Starters

You may not consider your slow cooker to be a great way to cook sides, but it's actually more useful than you might think. Dishes such as risotto, wild rice, and hearty grains are perfect for the slow cooker because you don't have to constantly stir or watch your pot.

Of course, even classics like potatoes and vegetables are great for the slow cooker because you can get them started while you're preparing a more complicated main dish. You won't use burners or oven space, and you can serve them directly from the pot.

Southern-Style Green Beans

SERVES 6

These slow-cooked green beans feature what you'd expect from Southern-style green beans, but with a twist. Whole garlic cloves give it an added depth of flavor, and the addition of chicken broth takes it up a notch. Make sure that you use fresh green beans for this dish. Canned will turn to mush in the cooker. Serve these tender beans with fried chicken, mashed potatoes, and gravy for a real Southern feast.

6 SLICES UNCOOKED BACON, CHOPPED
2 POUNDS FRESH GREEN BEANS, ENDS TRIMMED, CUT INTO 1-INCH PIECES
1 MEDIUM ONION, CHOPPED
1 CUP CHICKEN BROTH
4 CLOVES GARLIC, SMASHED
6 WHOLE BLACK PEPPERCORNS

Add all of the ingredients to slow cooker. Cover and cook on low heat for 6 hours until the beans are tender.

Before serving, remove the peppercorns and garlic cloves from the pot. Serve hot.

• Sides and Starters •

Orange-Glazed Carrots

SERVES 6

These are so easy, yet so delicious and a big hit at holiday dinners. The orange juice goes naturally with the sweetness of the honey and carrots, and is rounded out by the addition of thyme.

½ CUP BUTTER
¼ CUP HONEY
1 CUP ORANGE JUICE
1 TEASPOON DRIED THYME
½ CUP CHICKEN BROTH
2 POUNDS BABY CARROTS
SALT AND PEPPER, TO TASTE

Grease the inside of the slow cooker with cooking spray, butter, or oil.

Combine all of the ingredients in the slow cooker and stir to be sure the carrots are fully coated. Cover and cook on low for 4 to 6 hours until carrots are tender.

Serve hot.

Braised Root Vegetables

SERVES 6

If you've never had root vegetables that have been slow braised in a slow cooker, then you are in for a real treat. Sweet and creamy, they become full of earthy flavor when cooked low and slow in a slow cooker. Use any variety and combination of vegetables you want; just make sure that each piece is the same size so that they are all fully cooked when you serve them.

2 MEDIUM SWEET POTATOES, CUT INTO BITE-SIZED PIECES
3 LARGE CARROTS, CUT INTO BITE-SIZED PIECES
2 MEDIUM PARSNIPS, CUT INTO BITE-SIZED PIECES
2 MEDIUM RED ONIONS, QUARTERED
2 MEDIUM YUKON GOLD POTATOES, CUT INTO BITE-SIZED PIECES
½ CUP BUTTER, MELTED
½ CUP CHICKEN BROTH
1 TEASPOON DRIED THYME
SALT AND PEPPER, TO TASTE

Combine all of the ingredients in the slow cooker. Cover and cook on low for 4 to 5 hours or until the vegetables are tender.

Serve hot with the sauce spooned over the top.

Tomatoes, Corn, and Yellow Squash with Herbed Butter

SERVES 6

This dish is delicious any time of year, but it is particularly special in the summer when cherry tomatoes and corn are both super sweet and tasty. The addition of fresh summer herbs helps, as well. Of course, you can get all of these things at the grocery store any time of the year, so don't wait until the sun shines to make this fabulous side dish.

½ CUP BUTTER, MELTED
6 CUPS CORN
2 CUPS CHERRY TOMATOES
4 YELLOW SUMMER SQUASH, CUT INTO ½-INCH PIECES
SALT AND PEPPER, TO TASTE
2 TABLESPOONS CHOPPED FRESH HERBS (SUCH AS BASIL, CHIVES, PARSLEY, CILANTRO, OREGANO, DILL, OR A COMBINATION)

Combine the butter, corn, tomatoes, and squash in the slow cooker. Season with salt and pepper. Cover and cook on high for 2 hours, until the vegetables are tender.

Just before serving, stir in the fresh herbs.

Caribbean Black Beans

SERVES 8

Beans are the perfect things to cook in the slow cooker as they absorb flavors beautifully and benefit from the long cooking time. These island-spiced beans are great at a barbecues or with tacos at a Southwestern-themed dinner. Beans need to be covered with liquid throughout the cooking time, so you'll need to check periodically and add more liquid if necessary.

1 POUND DRIED BLACK BEANS, SOAKED OVERNIGHT
2 TABLESPOONS OLIVE OIL, OPTIONAL
2 MEDIUM ONIONS, CHOPPED
2 CLOVES GARLIC, CHOPPED
1 ANAHEIM CHILI PEPPER, SEEDED AND CHOPPED
1 MEDIUM RED BELL PEPPER, SEEDED AND CHOPPED
1 TEASPOON JERK SEASONING
1 BAY LEAF
5 CUPS CHICKEN BROTH
1 (14-OUNCE) CAN CRUSHED TOMATOES
2 TABLESPOONS LIME JUICE
SALT AND PEPPER, TO TASTE

Drain the beans, and add them to the slow cooker.

For deep flavor, sauté the onions, garlic, chili, and bell pepper along with the seasonings in the oil in a large skillet set over medium-high heat until tender, about 5 minutes. Transfer the vegetables to the slow cooker and add the broth, tomatoes, and lime juice. If you are pressed for time, simply combine the uncooked vegetables and seasonings with the beans, broth, tomatoes, and lime juice in the slow cooker and omit the oil. Season with salt and pepper.

Cover and cook on high for 5 hours, checking the liquid periodically. The beans will be tender and creamy when done.

Serve hot.

• Sides and Starters •

Roasted Beets with Pomegranate Dressing

SERVES 6

Beets are a controversial food for many people, as their bright color and strong earthiness can be a turnoff. If you're a beet hater but you've never had them roasted, you should try this recipe. Cooking them for a long period of time in the slow cooker brings out their natural sugars and makes them sweet, while toning down their raw flavor. Serve with the dressing atop field greens for a delicious main-dish salad or alongside roasted or grilled meats.

6 MEDIUM BEETS, SCRUBBED AND TRIMMED
1 CUP VEGETABLE OIL
½ CUP POMEGRANATE JUICE
¼ CUP RICE VINEGAR
2 SMALL SHALLOTS, FINELY CHOPPED
1 TABLESPOON SUGAR
SALT AND PEPPER, TO TASTE
8 OUNCES GOAT CHEESE, CRUMBLED, FOR GARNISH

Wrap each beet in aluminum foil, and put them in slow cooker. Cover and cook for 5 hours, until a knife inserted pierces the beets with no resistance.

Remove the beets from the cooker, unwrap, and allow them to cool completely. Peel the skins with a pairing knife.

Cut the cooled beets into wedges and put them in a bowl.

Whisk the oil, juice, vinegar, shallots, and sugar together and season with salt and pepper. Pour the dressing over the beets, and toss to coat.

Refrigerate for 2 hours to marinate. Serve chilled or at room temperature and garnish with the goat cheese.

Garlic and Rosemary Red Potatoes

SERVES 6

Cooked in olive oil infused with rosemary and garlic, these potatoes become sweet and tender when roasted for hours. These are great for holiday gatherings when you don't have space in the oven to roast potatoes to go alongside the meat. They require no chopping or prep; simply put whole red potatoes in the cooker with the rest of the ingredients and turn it on.

½ CUP OLIVE OIL
6 CLOVES GARLIC, SLICED
1 TABLESPOON CHOPPED FRESH ROSEMARY LEAVES
20 SMALL RED POTATOES
SALT AND PEPPER, TO TASTE

Combine the olive oil, garlic, rosemary, and potatoes in the slow cooker and stir until the potatoes are well coated with the oil. Season with salt and pepper.

Cover and cook on high for 4 hours.

Serve immediately.

• Sides and Starters •

Polenta

SERVES 6

Polenta is an Italian side dish that, if cooked on the stove, requires constant stirring to become creamy. Because of this intensive labor, there are many prepared products on the market, but none of them are nearly as tasty or authentic as a home-cooked version. With a slow cooker, all that changes, as you just put all of the ingredients into the pot and it does all the work.

6 CUPS CHICKEN BROTH OR WATER
2 CUPS CORNMEAL
4 TABLESPOONS BUTTER, CUT INTO SMALL PIECES
½ TEASPOON SALT

Grease the inside of the slow cooker with cooking spray, butter, or oil.

Combine the broth and cornmeal in the slow cooker, top with the butter, and add the salt.

Cover and cook on high for about 2 hours until polenta is smooth and creamy.

Serve hot.

Risotto alla Milanese

SERVES 6

There are a few things you have to know before you make risotto in the slow cooker. First of all, the type of rice matters. You need to get medium-grain rice labeled either arborio or carnaroli. These types of rice will produce the creamy and tender results you are looking for. The other thing to remember is that while the slow cooker will do all the hard work, you can't skip the step of cooking the rice in a little fat for a few minutes before transferring it to the slow cooker.

½ CUP BUTTER

2 TABLESPOONS OLIVE OIL

1 TEASPOON SAFFRON THREADS

2 MEDIUM SHALLOTS, CHOPPED

SALT AND PEPPER, TO TASTE

½ CUP ARBORIO OR CARNAROLI RICE

¼ CUP DRY WHITE WINE

4 CUPS CHICKEN OR VEGETABLE BROTH

½ CUP FRESHLY GRATED PARMESAN CHEESE, FOR GARNISH

Grease the inside of the slow cooker with cooking spray, butter, or oil.

Heat the butter and oil in a medium saucepan set over medium heat. Add the saffron and shallots and cook until the shallots are soft, about 5 minutes. Season with salt and pepper. Add the rice to the skillet and stir to coat with the oil. Cook until the rice begins to look opaque, about 2 minutes. Add the wine and continue to cook until the liquid evaporates.

Transfer the the contents of the saucepan to slow cooker and add the broth. Cover and cook on high for 2 hours. The risotto is done when the rice is tender and creamy.

Serve hot with more butter, if desired, and the cheese.

Saffron Rice

SERVES 6 TO 8

Saffron has a sublime flavor and will turn your dish bright yellow. You should buy it from a specialty retailer; if you purchase it from a local supermarket, you're going to get a lesser quality product and one that has likely been sitting on the shelves for too long.

2 TABLESPOONS BUTTER OR OLIVE OIL, OPTIONAL
2 SMALL SHALLOTS, CHOPPED
1 TEASPOON SAFFRON THREADS, CRUSHED
3 CUPS WHITE RICE
5 CUPS CHICKEN BROTH
2 CUPS PEAS

Grease the inside of the slow cooker with cooking spray, butter, or oil.

For deep flavor, sauté the shallots and saffron in the butter or olive oil in a medium skillet until the shallots are soft, about 5 minutes, and then add them to the slow cooker. If you are pressed for time, simply add the shallots and saffron to the slow cooker without pre-cooking, and omit the butter or oil.

Add the rice and broth to the slow cooker and stir to combine. Cover and cook on high for 2 hours until the rice is tender and the broth is absorbed. Just before serving, stir in the peas.

Serve hot.

Fruited Wild Rice Pilaf

SERVES 8

This particular dish makes an excellent stuffing for a pork roast or as a side dish to other roasted meats. Feel free to substitute the type of fruit and nuts you use. This recipe calls for apricots, cranberries, and almonds, but raisins, cherries, and plums work well, as do walnuts or pecans.

- 2 CUPS UNCOOKED WILD RICE
- 2 TABLESPOONS BUTTER OR OLIVE OIL, OPTIONAL
- 1 MEDIUM ONION, CHOPPED
- 3 CELERY STALKS, CHOPPED
- 5 CUPS CHICKEN OR VEGETABLE BROTH
- ½ CUP FINELY CHOPPED DRIED APRICOTS
- ½ CUP DRIED CRANBERRIES
- ½ CUP SLICED ALMONDS
- SALT AND PEPPER, TO TASTE

Grease the inside of the slow cooker with cooking spray, butter, or oil.

Add the rice to the slow cooker.

For deep flavor, sauté the onion and celery in the butter or olive oil until tender, about 5 minutes. Transfer the vegetables to the slow cooker. If you are pressed for time, simply add the onion and celery directly to the slow cooker without pre-cooking, and omit the butter or oil.

Add the broth and dried fruits to the slow cooker and stir to combine. Season with salt and pepper. Cover and cook on low for 7 hours or until the rice is tender, the fruit is plump, and the liquid is absorbed. Uncover and cook for an additional 30 minutes.

Just before serving, stir in the almonds. Serve hot.

Classic Bread Stuffing

SERVES 6 TO 8

Stuffing is a holiday staple at many dinner tables, whether it is stuffed into a bird or just eaten on the side. This is the classic recipe for stuffing filled with herbs and spices that immediately makes you think of the holidays. But now that you can cook it in the slow cooker, you can enjoy a taste of the holidays all year round.

6 CUPS STALE BREAD CRUMBS
½ CUP BUTTER
1 MEDIUM ONION, CHOPPED
2 CELERY STALKS, CHOPPED
2 TEASPOONS FINELY CHOPPED FRESH SAGE
2 TEASPOONS FINELY CHOPPED FRESH THYME
¼ CUP FINELY CHOPPED FRESH PARSLEY
SALT AND PEPPER, TO TASTE
3 CUPS CHICKEN BROTH
2 EGGS, BEATEN

Grease the inside of the slow cooker with cooking spray, butter, or oil.

Add the bread to the slow cooker.

Melt the butter in a medium skillet set over medium-high heat. Add the onion and celery and sauté until tender, about 5 minutes. Mix in the sage, thyme, parsley, salt, and pepper and transfer the mixture to the slow cooker.

Whisk the broth and eggs together in a bowl. Pour over the bread and vegetables in the slow cooker. Stir to combine.

Cover and cook on high for 1 hour, then turn the heat down to low. Cook for 5 hours until cooked through.

Serve hot.

Cornbread Stuffing

SERVES 6

This cornbread dressing is a tradition for many families around the holidays and for good reason. It's filled with salty and smoky ham, flavored with fresh herbs, and has bits of vegetables and fruit.

4 CUPS CRUMBLED STALE CORNBREAD
½ CUP BUTTER
1 MEDIUM ONION, CHOPPED
2 CELERY STALKS, CHOPPED
1 CUP DICED SMOKED HAM
SALT AND PEPPER, TO TASTE
¼ CUP CHOPPED FRESH HERBS
½ CUP CHOPPED DRIED APRICOTS
2 CUPS CHICKEN OR VEGETABLE BROTH
½ CUP MILK
1 EGG, BEATEN
4 DROPS HOT SAUCE

Grease the inside of the slow cooker with cooking spray, butter, or oil.

Add the cornbread to the slow cooker.

Melt the butter in a medium skillet set over medium-high heat. Add the onion, celery, and ham and sauté until the vegetables are tender, about 5 minutes. Season with salt and pepper and add the herbs. Transfer the mixture to the slow cooker, add the dried apricots, and stir to mix with the cornbread.

In a medium bowl, whisk together the broth, milk, egg, and hot sauce. Pour this mixture into the slow cooker and stir to mix.

Cover and cook on high for 1 hour. Reduce the heat to low and cook for 5 hours until cooked through.

Serve hot.

• Sides and Starters •

Vegetarian Cassoulet

SERVES 8

A cassoulet is a French casserole dish that is usually studded with several kinds of rich meats and beans simmered in a flavorful broth and then topped with crunchy bread crumbs. This version has no meat and is not nearly as time and labor intensive. (The traditional version can take several days to prepare!)

2 CUPS DRIED WHITE BEANS, SOAKED OVERNIGHT
½ CUP BROWN LENTILS
½ CUP SPLIT PEAS
¼ CUP OLIVE OIL, OPTIONAL
1 LARGE ONION, CHOPPED
5 CLOVES GARLIC, MINCED
4 MEDIUM CARROTS, CHOPPED
4 CELERY STALKS, CHOPPED
1 TEASPOON DRIED THYME
SALT AND PEPPER, TO TASTE
8 CUPS VEGETABLE BROTH
1 CUP RED WINE
1 (14-OUNCE) CAN CRUSHED TOMATOES
ZEST OF 1 ORANGE
1 BAY LEAF
1 CUP FRESH BREAD CRUMBS
½ CUP FRESHLY GRATED PARMESAN CHEESE
½ CUP CHOPPED PARSLEY

Grease the inside of the slow cooker with cooking spray, butter, or oil.

Add the beans, lentils, and peas to the slow cooker.

continued ▶

Vegetarian Cassoulet *continued* ▶

For deep flavor, heat the olive oil in a large skillet set over medium-high heat. Add the onion, garlic, carrots, and celery and sauté until the vegetables are tender, about 5 minutes. Stir in the thyme and season with salt and pepper. Transfer the mixture to the slow cooker. If you are pressed for time, simply add these ingredients to the cooker without pre-cooking, and omit the oil.

Add the broth, wine, tomatoes, orange zest, and bay leaf and stir to combine. Cover and cook on high for 5 hours until the beans are tender.

Remove the bay leaf from the pot. Combine the bread crumbs, Parmesan, and parsley in a small bowl. Sprinkle over the top of the casserole in an even layer. Cook uncovered for 30 minutes more.

Serve hot.

Eggplant Parmesan

SERVES 6

Eggplant is a perfect vegetable for the slow cooker. It has a meaty texture that takes beautifully to slow braising, and it absorbs the flavors of the seasonings it cooks in. Don't skip the step of salting the eggplant; if you do, you'll have a slow cooker filled with water.

1 LARGE EGGPLANT, CUT INTO ½-INCH ROUNDS
2 TABLESPOONS SALT, DIVIDED
1 (24-OUNCE) JAR MARINARA SAUCE
8 OUNCES FRESH MOZZARELLA CHEESE, SLICED
1 CUP FRESHLY GRATED PARMESAN CHEESE

Line a baking sheet with paper towels. Lay the eggplant rounds on the sheet and sprinkle them with 1 tablespoon of salt. Allow them to sit for 10 minutes. Turn the rounds over and sprinkle the other side with the remaining tablespoon of salt. Let them sit for 10 minutes more. Blot the eggplant with dry paper towels and set aside.

Grease the inside of the slow cooker with cooking spray, butter, or oil.

Spread a layer of the sauce on the bottom of the slow cooker and then top with a layer of eggplant. Add a layer of mozzarella and Parmesan cheeses. Top with more sauce, then another layer of eggplant, sauce, and another layer cheese. Repeat the layers until the cooker is three-quarters full or you have no ingredients left. The last layer should be cheese.

Cover and cook on low for 4 hours until the casserole is heated through and the cheese is bubbly.

Allow to rest for 10 minutes before serving.

Zucchini, Leek, and Tomato Gratin

SERVES 6

This delectable gratin is a great side dish. Do not skip the step of salting the tomatoes and zucchini; otherwise, you will end up with a soggy mess in the slow cooker.

4 CUPS ZUCCHINI, SHREDDED
3 TABLESPOONS SALT, DIVIDED
3 MEDIUM TOMATOES, SLICED
4 TABLESPOONS OLIVE OIL, DIVIDED
2 LEEKS, WHITE AND LIGHT GREEN PARTS, SLICED
½ CUP VEGETABLE BROTH
2 TABLESPOONS TOMATO PASTE
2 TEASPOONS CHOPPED FRESH TARRAGON
FRESHLY GRATED PARMESAN, FOR GARNISH

Put the zucchini in a colander and sprinkle liberally with 1 tablespoon of salt. Press down on it to drain any excess moisture. Set aside. Arrange the tomato slices on paper towels and sprinkle with 1 tablespoon of salt. Turn the tomato slices over and sprinkle the other side with the remaining tablespoon of salt. Set aside.

Put 2 tablespoons of oil in the bottom of the slow cooker. Toss the leeks with the remaining 2 tablespoons of oil and set aside.

In a small bowl, combine the broth, tomato paste, and tarragon.

Layer some of the tomatoes on the bottom of the slow cooker and drizzle with some of the broth mixture. Add a layer of zucchini and another layer of the broth mixture. Add some of the leeks and another layer of the broth mixture. Continue to layer the ingredients in this order until the pot is three-quarters full or you have no ingredients left. The top layer should be the broth mixture.

Cover and cook on high for about 2 hours until the vegetables are tender. Remove the cover, and cook on low for another hour.

Serve the gratin at room temperature sprinkled with the Parmesan cheese.

Ratatouille with Goat Cheese and Basil

SERVES 4 TO 6

Ratatouille is a classic tomato-y French stew of summer vegetables, including eggplant and squash. The key to getting the right consistency in the slow cooker is to slice the vegetables as thinly as possible. A mandolin slicer is fast and consistent, but a sharp knife and steady hand will do. Serve this with couscous and top with the creamy goat cheese and fresh basil for a fast, healthful, and super delicious weeknight meal.

1 LARGE EGGPLANT, THINLY SLICED
2 LARGE RED BELL PEPPERS, THINLY SLICED
2 SMALL ZUCCHINI, THINLY SLICED
1 RED ONION, THINLY SLICED
1 YELLOW SQUASH, THINLY SLICED
SALT AND PEPPER, TO TASTE
1 (32-OUNCE) JAR MARINARA SAUCE
2 TABLESPOONS OLIVE OIL
8 OUNCES GOAT CHEESE, CRUMBLED, FOR GARNISH
½ CUP SLICED FRESH BASIL, FOR GARNISH

Grease the inside of the slow cooker with cooking spray, butter, or oil.

Layer the vegetables in alternating layers in the slow cooker until they are gone or the pot is three-quarters full. Season with salt and pepper.

Pour the sauce and oil over the vegetables, cover, and cook on low for 7 to 8 hours until the vegetables are tender.

To serve, spoon over couscous, rice, or pasta, and garnish with the goat cheese and fresh basil.

Italian Cocktail Meatballs

MAKES ABOUT 24 MEATBALLS

These meatballs make great appetizers or you can serve them with buns for easy meatball subs. These meatballs are made of beef and pork and cook up to tender perfection in the slow cooker.

4 PIECES SOFT WHITE BREAD, TORN
1 CUP MILK
1 POUND LEAN GROUND BEEF
1 POUND BULK ITALIAN SAUSAGE
1 POUND LEAN GROUND PORK
1 MEDIUM ONION, CHOPPED
½ CUP CHOPPED FRESH PARSLEY
1 CUP FRESHLY GRATED PARMESAN CHEESE
3 EGGS
PINCH OF NUTMEG
1 (32-OUNCE) JAR OF YOUR FAVORITE PASTA SAUCE

Grease the inside of the slow cooker with cooking spray, butter, or oil.

Put the bread and milk in a large bowl and let the bread sit until the milk is absorbed. Add the beef, sausage, pork, onion, parsley, cheese, eggs, and nutmeg and mix, using your hands, until just combined, being careful not to over mix.

Place the sauce in the slow cooker. Using your hands or a scoop, form the meat mixture into 1-inch meatballs and add them to the pot. Cover and cook on high for 1 hour.

Reduce heat to low and cook for 3 more hours until the meatballs register at 165 degrees F on an instant-read thermometer.

Serve the meatballs hot over pasta or rolls, if desired.

• Sides and Starters •

Asian Honey Chicken Wings

SERVES 8

Wings are popular entertaining food. With the slow cooker, they're also easy to cook and easy to serve. You'll definitely want to brown the wings before adding them to the cooker, as this adds to their flavor and crisp texture.

3 POUNDS CHICKEN WINGS
¼ CUP OLIVE OIL
1 TEASPOON PAPRIKA
½ TEASPOON SALT
½ TEASPOON PEPPER
1 CUP HONEY
½ CUP SOY SAUCE
½ CUP HOISIN SAUCE
¼ CUP RICE WINE
2 CLOVES GARLIC, FINELY CHOPPED
1 TEASPOON MINCED FRESH GINGER

Grease the inside of the slow cooker with cooking spray, butter, or oil.

Preheat the broiler to high. Put the wings, oil, paprika, salt, and pepper in a large bowl and toss to coat. Transfer the wings to a baking sheet and broil them for 5 minutes until crispy. Turn them over and broil the other side for 5 minutes.

In the slow cooker, combine the honey, soy sauce, hoisin sauce, rice wine, garlic, and ginger. Add the wings and toss to coat. Cover and cook for about 3 hours, stirring once or twice to ensure that the wings are thoroughly coated and cooking evenly.

Serve hot and coated in the sauce.

Super Bowl Chili

SERVES 10

Chili is the perfect dish for slow cooker cooking. There are many variations, but this one is a classic spicy version made with beef ribs. Don't forget condiments: sour cream, cheese, jalapeños, and hot sauce make this dish Super Bowl worthy. This recipe makes enough to feed a crowd, so you'll need a five- to seven-quart slow cooker.

2 TABLESPOONS VEGETABLE OIL, DIVIDED
1 LARGE ONION, CHOPPED
1 JALAPEÑO PEPPER, SEEDED AND CHOPPED
1 TEASPOON ANCHO CHILI POWDER
2 TO 3 POUNDS BONELESS BEEF RIBS, CUT INTO BITE-SIZED PIECES
3 CUPS BEEF BROTH
1 (32-OUNCE) CAN CRUSHED TOMATOES AND THEIR JUICES
2 (14-OUNCE) CANS PINTO BEANS, RINSED AND DRAINED
CONDIMENTS OF YOUR CHOICE

Grease the inside of the slow cooker with cooking spray, butter, or oil.

Heat half the oil in a large skillet over medium-high heat. Add the onion and jalapeño and sauté until the onion is soft, about 4 minutes. Stir in the chili powder and cook for another minute. Transfer the mixture to the slow cooker.

In the same skillet, add the remaining oil and the meat. Cook, turning several times, until the meat is browned on all sides. Transfer the meat to the slow cooker.

Add the broth, tomatoes and juice, and beans to the slow cooker and stir to mix. Cover and cook on low for about 10 hours or until the beef is tender and the chili has thickened.

Serve the chili hot from the slow cooker with desired garnishes.

CHAPTER NINE

Desserts and Drinks

CHAPTER NINE

Desserts and Drinks

If you'd rather come home to the smell of vanilla or baked fruit instead of more savory fare, the slow cooker is the way to go. From hot fudge cake to hot cocoa, you'll be amazed at the mouthwatering desserts and drinks you can whip up, all in one pot.

And, making treats in a slow cooker is pretty foolproof. For the most part, you're just going to add the ingredients to the pot and let it cook until it's done. No scientific methods, buying specific thermometers, or worrying about humidity.

Strawberry Rhubarb White Chocolate Crumble

SERVES 8

This dish is best made in the early spring when rhubarb is in season and strawberries are at their peak. When you combine the oats and white chocolate, you'll have a classic dessert with a slight twist that is perfect served warm from the pot with some vanilla ice cream.

4 CUPS STRAWBERRIES, HULLED AND QUARTERED
4 RHUBARB STALKS, CUT INTO ½-INCH PIECES
2 CUPS SUGAR
1 TEASPOON CINNAMON
ZEST OF 1 ORANGE
1 TABLESPOON CORNSTARCH
1 CUP ROLLED OATS (NOT INSTANT)
1 CUP FLOUR
½ CUP (PACKED) LIGHT BROWN SUGAR
½ CUP CHOPPED WHITE CHOCOLATE
½ CUP BUTTER, CHILLED

Grease the inside of the slow cooker with cooking spray, butter, or oil.

In the slow cooker, combine the strawberries, rhubarb, sugar, cinnamon, and zest.

To make the crumble, combine the cornstarch, oats, flour, brown sugar, and white chocolate in a medium bowl. Add the cold butter and, using either your fingers or two knives, cut the butter into the mixture until it turns into a pea-sized crumble. Sprinkle the crumble mixture over the fruit in the slow cooker.

Cover and cook on low for 2 to 3 hours until the crumble is set and the fruit is bubbling.

Before serving, uncover the pot and allow the crumble to cool for about 30 minutes.

Serve warm with vanilla ice cream.

Spiced Pear Crumble

SERVES 8

The slow cooker is great for rustic fruit desserts such as this pear crumble that is studded with almonds and flavored with amaretto. When choosing pears for this dish, you want to select those that are firm, as softer fruit will disintegrate when cooked for a long period of time. You can serve this fragrant dish with vanilla ice cream or a dollop of whipped cream.

1 CUP (PACKED) BROWN SUGAR
¾ CUP BUTTER, MELTED, DIVIDED
¼ CUP AMARETTO LIQUEUR
8 LARGE FIRM PEARS, PEELED, CORED, AND CHOPPED
½ CUP SUGAR
½ CUP FLOUR
½ CUP SLICED ALMONDS, TOASTED
1 TEASPOON CINNAMON
¼ TEASPOON NUTMEG

Grease the inside of the slow cooker with cooking spray, butter, or oil.

In the slow cooker, combine the brown sugar, ½ cup of butter, and the amaretto. Add the pears and stir to coat.

In a small bowl, combine the sugar, flour, almonds, cinnamon, nutmeg, and the remaining ¼ cup of butter. Stir with a fork until it starts to clump. Sprinkle this mixture over the pears in the slow cooker.

Cover and cook on high for 3 hours or until a toothpick inserted in the center comes out clean. Remove the lid and allow to cool for about 30 minutes.

Serve warm.

Apple Cranberry Cobbler

SERVES 8

Apples and cranberries are a classic fall combination and pair beautifully in this slow-cooked cobbler flavored with maple syrup. You can use any type of firm baking apple in this dish, but Golden Delicious go perfectly with the tart cranberries. This cobbler is fabulous when served warm with a scoop of vanilla ice cream.

5 OR 6 LARGE GOLDEN DELICIOUS APPLES, OR THE VARIETY OF YOUR CHOICE, PEELED, CORED, AND CHOPPED
12 OUNCES FRESH CRANBERRIES
2 CUPS SUGAR, DIVIDED
1 TABLESPOON CORNSTARCH
1 TEASPOON CINNAMON
1 TEASPOON GROUND CLOVES
¼ TEASPOON GROUND GINGER
1½ CUPS BUTTER, MELTED
2 CUPS FLOUR
¼ CUP MAPLE SYRUP
2 EGGS, BEATEN

Grease the inside of the slow cooker with cooking spray, butter, or oil.

In the slow cooker, combine the apples, cranberries, 1 cup of sugar, cornstarch, cinnamon, cloves, and ginger.

In a medium bowl, mix the butter, flour, the remaining sugar, maple syrup, and eggs. Pour the mixture into the slow cooker. Cover and cook on high for 2 hours or until a toothpick inserted in the center comes out clean.

Uncover and allow to cool for 30 minutes.

Serve warm.

Hot Fudge Cake

SERVES 6

If you love rich desserts but don't want to spend the time learning the scientific process of baking them, then you will love this slow cooker hot fudge cake. This is a surprisingly simple recipe that will never let you down. The top layer is a tender and moist chocolate cake, while the bottom layer is a delicious cross between rich hot fudge sauce and creamy chocolate pudding. When using cocoa powder for this cake, be sure to select natural and not Dutch process.

½ CUP MILK
3 TABLESPOONS BUTTER, MELTED
1 TEASPOON PURE VANILLA EXTRACT
1 CUP SUGAR
1 CUP FLOUR
½ CUP UNSWEETENED COCOA POWDER, DIVIDED
1 TABLESPOON BAKING POWDER
¾ CUP PACKED BROWN SUGAR
1½ CUPS BOILING WATER

Grease the inside of the slow cooker with cooking spray, butter, or oil.

In a mixing bowl, combine the milk, butter, and vanilla. Slowly add in the sugar, flour, ¼ cup cocoa powder, and the baking powder. Spread the batter in the bottom of the slow cooker.

In a medium bowl, mix together the brown sugar and remaining cocoa powder. Sprinkle this evenly over the batter in the slow cooker. Pour the boiling water into the cooker, and do not stir.

Cover and cook on high heat for 2 hours or until a toothpick inserted in the center comes out clean.

Uncover and allow to cool for 20 minutes.

Serve with vanilla ice cream or whipped cream.

Chocolate Croissant Bread Pudding

SERVES 6 TO 8

What could be better than warm, melted chocolate flecked throughout flaky and buttery croissants? After you've tasted this, you'll agree that nothing much beats this bread pudding. Serve this with fresh berries or vanilla ice cream for a dessert you'll come back to again and again.

6 LARGE CROISSANTS, PREFERABLY A DAY OLD
4 OUNCES SEMISWEET CHOCOLATE, CHOPPED, DIVIDED
4 TABLESPOONS BUTTER, MELTED
6 LARGE EGGS
2 CUPS HEAVY CREAM
½ CUP SUGAR
1 TABLESPOON PURE VANILLA EXTRACT

Grease the inside of the slow cooker with cooking spray, butter, or oil.

Tear the croissants into bite-sized pieces, and add them to the slow cooker. Sprinkle with half of the chopped chocolate.

Melt the butter with the remaining chocolate in the microwave or a small saucepan and allow it to cool completely.

Beat the eggs with the cream, sugar, and vanilla. Add the melted chocolate. Pour this mixture over the croissants, making sure that all of the pieces are submerged in liquid.

Cover and cook on high for about 3 hours until the bread pudding has puffed up. Remove the lid and allow to cool for about 20 minutes before serving.

• Desserts and Drinks •

Tapioca Pudding

SERVES 6 TO 8

The difference between store-bought tapioca pudding and homemade is amazing. When you buy it from the supermarket, the texture may be off and the flavor may be artificial or just plain bland. This slow cooker version is anything but. It's creamy and rich with hints of vanilla and pure cream. It's a great comforting dessert that will cure the blues on a gray day.

3 CUPS WHOLE MILK
1½ CUPS SUGAR
1 CUP HEAVY CREAM
½ CUP PEARL TAPIOCA
2 EGGS
ZEST OF 1 ORANGE
1 TABLESPOON PURE VANILLA EXTRACT

Grease the inside of the slow cooker with cooking spray, butter, or oil.

In the slow cooker, whisk together the milk, sugar, and cream. Sprinkle the tapioca over the top.

Cover and cook on low heat for about 2 hours until the tapioca is transparent.

In a small bowl, combine the eggs eggs, orange zest, and vanilla extract. Beat until combined.

Stir this mixture into the pudding mixture in the slow cooker.

Cover and cook for another 30 to 40 minutes until the milk is fully absorbed.

Take off the lid and allow the pudding to cool for 30 minutes.

Serve warm or chilled.

Wassail

SERVES 12

There are many variations of wassail. Some are made with apple cider, while others are made with beer or wine. This version is made with wine for an adults-only treat that brings a festive fall aroma to any gathering. The smell of mulled wine and spices will fill your house with the natural scents of cloves, oranges, and anise.

1 ORANGE
15 TO 20 WHOLE CLOVES
THREE BOTTLES RED WINE, SUCH AS ZINFANDEL OR PINOT NOIR
2 CUPS DRIED APPLE SLICES
1 CUP SUGAR
3 STAR ANISE PODS
1 SMALL LEMON, SLICED, SEEDS REMOVED

Without peeling the orange, stud it with the cloves. Add it to the slow cooker.

Add the wine, apples, sugar, star anise, and lemon slices to the slow cooker. Cover and cook on low for 3 to 4 hours.

Strain the wassail, or simply remove everything except the lemon slices with a slotted spoon.

Serve warm from the slow cooker.

Warmed Cranberry Punch

SERVES 12

In addition to the holiday flavor of this fruity, spiced punch, the aroma will put your guests in a festive mood. When you serve this right from the slow cooker, guests can help themselves and each cup will be at the perfect serving temperature. This means you can worry about more important things than whether everyone has the desired drink in hand.

6 CUPS CRANBERRY JUICE
4 CUPS PINEAPPLE JUICE
1 CUP WATER
½ CUP SUGAR
3 CINNAMON STICKS
1 TEASPOON WHOLE CLOVES
½ TEASPOON WHOLE ALLSPICE

Combine all of the ingredients in the slow cooker. Cover and cook for about 2 hours.

Remove the whole spices before serving.

Serve warm from the slow cooker.

White Chocolate Mocha

SERVES 12

This makes a nice treat at a holiday party or a midwinter brunch. When choosing white chocolate for this warm concoction, be sure to use a bar instead of chips. The chips may be waxy in texture and might not melt completely, leaving some guests thinking that they have small pebbles in their drinks. Top with whipped cream, chocolate shavings, or even finely chopped peppermints if the mood strikes.

2 CUPS WHOLE MILK
2 CUPS HEAVY CREAM
1 POUND WHITE CHOCOLATE BAR, FINELY CHOPPED OR GRATED
8 CUPS STRONGLY BREWED COFFEE
1 TABLESPOON PURE VANILLA EXTRACT

Put the milk, cream, and white chocolate in a saucepan and heat over medium heat until the chocolate is melted and smooth.

Pour the mixture into the slow cooker and add the coffee and vanilla.

Cover and cook on low for 2 to 3 hours. Turn the cooker down to warm, and serve directly from the cooker.

Creamy Hot Cocoa

SERVES 10

While it can be difficult to serve this from the slow cooker, this version never fails to be creamy, hot, and delicious from the first serving to the last. Set out lots of garnishes such as marshmallows, sprinkles, crushed peppermint candies, and shaved chocolate for a festive treat both kids and adults will love.

4 CUPS WHOLE MILK
2 CUPS HEAVY CREAM
1 POUND SEMI-SWEET CHOCOLATE, CHOPPED
1 TABLESPOON PURE VANILLA EXTRACT

Combine all of the ingredients in the slow cooker. Cover and cook on low for about 1 hour. Remove the lid and stir the chocolate with a whisk to get all the melted chocolate off the bottom of the pot. Cover and cook on low for another hour. Remove the lid, stir, and reduce the heat to warm.

Serve warm from the slow cooker.

Index

A
American favorites, 35–44
    Barbecued Baby Back Ribs, 40
    Chicken Potpie, 43
    Classic Pot Roast, 44
    Franks and Beans, 42
    Old-Fashioned Beef Stew, 36
    Old-Fashioned Meatloaf, 39
    Pork Chops with Apples and Sauerkraut, 41
    Pulled-Pork Barbecue, 38
    Shredded Buffalo Chicken, 37
Apples
    Apple Cranberry Cobbler, 108
    Curried Coconut Chicken with Basil, 53
    Pork Chops with Apples and Sauerkraut, 41
Apricots
    Chicken and Mushroom Casserole, 78
    Cornbread Stuffing, 94
    Fruited Wild Rice Pilaf, 92
    Moroccan Chicken Tagine, 49
    North African Beef Stew, 51
Artichoke hearts
    Poached Salmon Cakes with White Wine Butter Sauce, 67
    Salmon, Artichoke, and Noodle Casserole, 77
Asian Honey Chicken Wings, 101

B
Bacon
    Franks and Beans, 42
    Southern-Style Green Beans, 82
    Veal Paprikash, 55
Baked Potato Soup, 22
Barbecued Baby Back Ribs, 40
Basil
    Curried Coconut Chicken with Basil, 53
    Ratatouille with Goat Cheese and Basil, 99
Beef
    Barbecued Baby Back Ribs, 40
    Braised Asian Beef, 57
    Classic Pot Roast, 44
    North African Beef Stew, 51
    Old-Fashioned Beef Stew, 36
    Super Bowl Chili, 102
Beets
    Roasted Beets with Pomegranate Dressing, 87
Bell pepper
    Caribbean Black Beans, 86
    Old-Fashioned Meatloaf, 39
    Ratatouille with Goat Cheese and Basil, 99
    Spicy Chicken Tortilla Soup, 30
    Veal Paprikash, 55
Black beans
    Caribbean Black Beans, 86
Bouillabaisse, 62–63
Braised Asian Beef, 57
Braised Root Vegetables, 84
Bread crumbs
    Classic Bread Stuffing, 93
    Vegetarian Cassoulet, 95–96
Bread pieces
    Classic Strata, 14
    Italian Cocktail Meatballs, 100
Breakfast, 13–17
    Classic Strata, 14
    Sausage and Potato Casserole, 15
    Slow Cooker Oatmeal, 17
    Spicy Pears with Cranberries, 16
Broccoli
    Cream of Broccoli Soup, 26
    Miso Chicken with Broccoli, 50
Butternut squash
    Slow-Cooked Butternut Squash Soup, 24

C
Caribbean Black Beans, 86
Carrots
    Braised Root Vegetables, 84
    Chicken Potpie, 43
    Classic Pot Roast, 44
    North African Beef Stew, 51
    Old-Fashioned Beef Stew, 36
    Orange-Glazed Carrots, 83
    Osso Bucco, 52
    Vegetarian Cassoulet, 95–96
Casseroles, 73–78
    Chicken and Mushroom Casserole, 78
    Classic Lasagna Bolognese, 75–76
    Salmon, Artichoke, and Noodle Casserole, 77
    Sausage and Potato Casserole, 15
    Tuna Noodle Casserole, 74
    Vegetarian Cassoulet, 95–96
Celery
    Fruited Wild Rice Pilaf, 92
    Hearty Bean Soup, 28
    Slow-Cooked Butternut Squash Soup, 24
    Tuna Noodle Casserole, 74
    Vegetarian Cassoulet, 95–96

Index

Cheddar cheese
    Classic Strata, 14
    Sausage and Potato Casserole, 15
Cherry tomatoes
    Tomatoes, Corn, and Yellow Squash with Herbed Butter, 85
Chicken
    Asian Honey Chicken Wings, 101
    Chicken and Mushroom Casserole, 78
    Chicken and Wild Rice Soup, 29
    Chicken Potpie, 43
    Curried Coconut Chicken with Basil, 53
    Miso Chicken with Broccoli, 50
    Moroccan Chicken Tagine, 49
    Shredded Buffalo Chicken, 37
    Spicy Chicken Tortilla Soup, 30
    Tandoori Chicken, 48
Chili
    Super Bowl Chili, 102
Chili pepper
    Caribbean Black Beans, 86
Chocolate
    Chocolate Croissant Bread Pudding, 110
    Creamy Hot Cocoa, 115
    Hot Fudge Cake, 109
    Strawberry Rhubarb White Chocolate Crumble, 106
    White Chocolate Mocha, 114
Clams
    Bouillabaisse, 62–63
Classic Bread Stuffing, 93
Classic Pot Roast, 44
Coconut milk
    Curried Coconut Chicken with Basil, 53
    Green Curried Shrimp, 69–70
Cod
    Sweet Miso-Glazed Cod, 66
Coffee
    White Chocolate Mocha, 114
Corn
    Chicken Potpie, 43
    Mexican-Style Pork, 56
    Old-Fashioned Beef Stew, 36
    Summer Vegetable Soup, 31
    Tomatoes, Corn, and Yellow Squash with Herbed Butter, 85

Cornbread Stuffing, 94
Cornmeal
    Polenta, 89
Cranberries
    Apple Cranberry Cobbler, 108
    Fruited Wild Rice Pilaf, 92
    Spicy Pears with Cranberries, 16
    Warmed Cranberry Punch, 113
Cream of Broccoli Soup, 26
Crock Pot, differences between slow cooker and, 4
Croissants
    Chocolate Croissant Bread Pudding, 110
Curried Coconut Chicken with Basil, 53

D
Desserts, 106–111
    Apple Cranberry Cobbler, 108
    Chocolate Croissant Bread Pudding, 110
    Hot Fudge Cake, 109
    Spiced Pear Crumble, 107
    Strawberry Rhubarb White Chocolate Crumble, 106
    Tapioca Pudding, 111
Dried Beans
    Hearty Bean Soup, 28
Drinks, 112–115
    Creamy Hot Cocoa, 114
    Warmed Cranberry Punch, 113
    Wassail, 112
    White Chocolate Mocha, 114

E
Eggplant
    Eggplant Parmesan, 97
    Ratatouille with Goat Cheese and Basil, 99
Eggs
    Classic Strata, 14
    Sausage and Potato Casserole, 15

F
Fish and seafood, 61–70
    Bouillabaisse, 62–63
    Green Curried Shrimp, 69–70
    Lemon and Garlic Halibut, 65
    Poached Salmon Cakes with White Wine Butter Sauce, 67
    Poached Tuna, 64

    Sea Bass with Spicy Crusted Potatoes, 68
    Sweet Miso-Glazed Cod, 66
Franks and Beans, 42
Fruited Wild Rice Pilaf, 92

G
Garbanzo beans
    North African Beef Stew, 51
Garlic and Rosemary Red Potatoes, 88
Goat cheese
    Ratatouille with Goat Cheese and Basil, 99
    Roasted Beets with Pomegranate Dressing, 87
Green beans
    Mediterranean Lamb, 58
    Southern-Style Green Beans, 82
    Summer Vegetable Soup, 31
Green Curried Shrimp, 69–70
Ground beef
    Classic Lasagna Bolognese, 75–76
    Italian Cocktail Meatballs, 100
    Old-Fashioned Meatloaf, 39

H
Halibut
    Bouillabaisse, 62–63
    Lemon and Garlic Halibut, 65
Ham
    Cornbread Stuffing, 94
    Ham and White Bean Soup, 27
    Hearty Bean Soup, 28
Hearty Bean Soup, 28
Heavy cream
    Roasted Tomato Soup, 25
Hot dogs
    Franks and Beans, 42
Hot Fudge Cake, 109

I
International dishes, 47–58
    Bouillabaisse, 62–63
    Braised Asian Beef, 57
    Curried Coconut Chicken with Basil, 53
    Green Curried Shrimp, 69–70
    Italian Cocktail Meatballs, 100
    Kielbasa and Sauerkraut, 54
    Mediterranean Lamb, 58
    Mexican-Style Pork, 56

Index

Miso Chicken with Broccoli, 50
Moroccan Chicken Tagine, 49
North African Beef Stew, 51
Osso Bucco, 52
Ratatouille with Goat Cheese and Basil, 99
Risotto alla Milanese, 90
Tandoori Chicken, 48
Veal Paprikash, 55
Vegetarian Cassoulet, 95–96
Italian Cocktail Meatballs, 100
Italian sausage
  Italian Cocktail Meatballs, 100

K
Kielbasa and Sauerkraut, 54

L
Lamb
  Mediterranean Lamb, 58
Lasagna
  Classic Lasagna Bolognese, 75–76
Leeks
  Baked Potato Soup, 22
  Bouillabaisse, 62–63
  Zucchini, Leek, and Tomato Gratin, 98
Lemon and Garlic Halibut, 65
Lemongrass
  Green Curried Shrimp, 69–70
Lentils
  Vegetarian Cassoulet, 95–96

M
Mediterranean Lamb, 58
Mexican-Style Pork, 56
Miso Chicken with Broccoli, 50
Moroccan Chicken Tagine, 49
Mozzarella cheese
  Classic Lasagna Bolognese, 75–76
  Eggplant Parmesan, 97
Multi-Mushroom Soup, 23
Mushrooms
  Chicken and Mushroom Casserole, 78
  Chicken and Wild Rice Soup, 29
  Multi-Mushroom Soup, 23
  Tuna Noodle Casserole, 74
Mussels
  Bouillabaisse, 62–63

N
Noodles
  Salmon, Artichoke, and Noodle Casserole, 77
  Tuna Noodle Casserole, 74
North African Beef Stew, 51

O
Oatmeal
  Slow Cooker Oatmeal, 17
Old-Fashioned Beef Stew, 36
Old-Fashioned Meatloaf, 39
Onions
  Braised Root Vegetables, 84
  Classic Pot Roast, 44
  North African Beef Stew, 51
  Old-Fashioned Beef Stew, 36
  Old-Fashioned Meatloaf, 39
Orange
  Orange-Glazed Carrots, 83
  Wassail, 112
Osso Bucco, 52

P
Parsnips
  Braised Root Vegetables, 84
Pears
  Spiced Pear Crumble, 107
  Spicy Pears with Cranberries, 16
Peas
  Chicken Potpie, 43
  Old-Fashioned Beef Stew, 36
Pineapple
  Warmed Cranberry Punch, 113
Pinto beans
  Super Bowl Chili, 102
Plums
  Moroccan Chicken Tagine, 49
Poached Salmon Cakes with White Wine Butter Sauce, 67
Poached Tuna, 64
Polenta, 89
Pomegranates
  Roasted Beets with Pomegranate Dressing, 87
Pork. *See also* Ham
  Classic Lasagna Bolognese, 75–76
  Italian Cocktail Meatballs, 100
  Mexican-Style Pork, 56
  Pork Chops with Apples and Sauerkraut, 41
  Pulled-Pork Barbecue, 38

Potatoes
  Baked Potato Soup, 22
  Braised Root Vegetables, 84
  Chicken Potpie, 43
  Classic Pot Roast, 44
  Garlic and Rosemary Red Potatoes, 88
  Mediterranean Lamb, 58
  Old-Fashioned Beef Stew, 36
  Sausage and Potato Casserole, 15
  Sea Bass with Spicy Crusted Potatoes, 68
  Summer Vegetable Soup, 31
Pulled-Pork Barbecue, 38

R
Ratatouille with Goat Cheese and Basil, 99
Red wine
  Wassail, 112
Rhubarb
  Strawberry Rhubarb White Chocolate Crumble, 106
Rice. *See* Wild rice
  Risotto alla Milanese, 90
  Saffron Rice, 91
Ricotta cheese
  Roasted Tomato Soup, 25
Risotto alla Milanese, 90
Roasted Beets with Pomegranate Dressing, 87
Roasted Tomato Soup, 25
Rosemary
  Garlic and Rosemary Red Potatoes, 88

S
Saffron Rice, 91
Salmon
  Poached Salmon Cakes with White Wine Butter Sauce, 67
  Salmon, Artichoke, and Noodle Casserole, 77
Sauerkraut
  Kielbasa and Sauerkraut, 54
  Pork Chops with Apples and Sauerkraut, 41
Sausage and Potato Casserole, 15
Sea Bass with Spicy Crusted Potatoes, 68
Shredded Buffalo Chicken, 37

Index

Shrimp
  Green Curried Shrimp, 69–70
Sides, 81–102
  Braised Root Vegetables, 84
  Caribbean Black Beans, 86
  Classic Bread Stuffing, 93
  Cornbread Stuffing, 94
  Eggplant Parmesan, 97
  Fruited Wild Rice Pilaf, 92
  Garlic and Rosemary Red Potatoes, 88
  Orange-Glazed Carrots, 83
  Polenta, 89
  Ratatouille with Goat Cheese and Basil, 99
  Risotto alla Milanese, 90
  Roasted Beets with Pomegranate Dressing, 87
  Saffron Rice, 91
  Southern-Style Green Beans, 82
  Tomatoes, Corn, and Yellow Squash with Herbed Butter, 85
  Vegetarian Cassoulet, 95–96
  Zucchini, Leek, and Tomato Gratin, 98
Slow-Cooked Butternut Squash Soup, 24
Slow Cooker Oatmeal, 17
Slow cookers
  basics of, 4
  basics of pantry for, 5–7
  differences between Crock Pots and, 4
  lid for, 8
  methods of cooking, 7
  order of ingredients and, 8
  settings on, 8
  sizes of, 8
  tips for, 8–9
  types of cooking in, 4–5
Soups, 21–31
  Baked Potato Soup, 22
  Chicken and Wild Rice Soup, 29
  Cream of Broccoli Soup, 26
  Ham and White Bean Soup, 27
  Hearty Bean Soup, 28
  Multi-Mushroom Soup, 23
  Roasted Tomato Soup, 25
  Slow-Cooked Butternut Squash Soup, 24
  Spicy Chicken Tortilla Soup, 30
  Summer Vegetable Soup, 31
Southern-Style Green Beans, 82
Spiced Pear Crumble, 107
Spicy Chicken Tortilla Soup, 30
Spicy Pears with Cranberries, 16
Squash. *See also* Butternut squash
  Ratatouille with Goat Cheese and Basil, 99
  Tomatoes, Corn, and Yellow Squash with Herbed Butter, 85
Starters
  Asian Honey Chicken Wings, 101
  Italian Cocktail Meatballs, 100
  Super Bowl Chili, 102
Strawberry Rhubarb White Chocolate Crumble, 106
Stuffing
  Classic Bread Stuffing, 93
  Cornbread Stuffing, 94
Summer Vegetable Soup, 31
Super Bowl Chili, 102
Sweet Miso-Glazed Cod, 66
Sweet potatoes
  Braised Root Vegetables, 84

T

Tandoori Chicken, 48
Tapioca Pudding, 111
Tomatoes. *See also* Cherry tomatoes
  Bouillabaisse, 62–63
  Caribbean Black Beans, 86
  Classic Lasagna Bolognese, 75–76
  Ham and White Bean Soup, 27
  Hearty Bean Soup, 28
  Roasted Tomato Soup, 25
  Spicy Chicken Tortilla Soup, 30
  Super Bowl Chili, 102
  Tomatoes, Corn, and Yellow Squash with Herbed Butter, 85
  Veal Paprikash, 55
  Vegetarian Cassoulet, 95–96
  Zucchini, Leek, and Tomato Gratin, 98
Tuna
  Poached Tuna, 64
  Tuna Noodle Casserole, 74

V

Veal
  Classic Lasagna Bolognese, 75–76
  Osso Bucco, 52
  Veal Paprikash, 55
Vegetarian Cassoulet, 95–96

W

White beans
  Franks and Beans, 42
  Ham and White Bean Soup, 27
  Vegetarian Cassoulet, 95–96
Wild rice
  Chicken and Mushroom Casserole, 78
  Chicken and Wild Rice Soup, 29
  Fruited Wild Rice Pilaf, 92

Y

Yogurt
  Tandoori Chicken, 48

Z

Zucchini
  Ratatouille with Goat Cheese and Basil, 99
  Zucchini, Leek, and Tomato Gratin, 98

Made in the USA
Lexington, KY
16 February 2014